The Aromatherapy Workbook

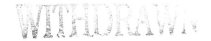

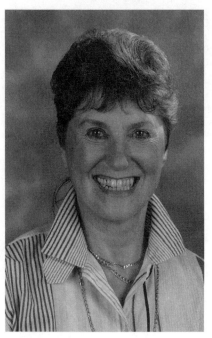

About the Author

Shirley Price has been a practising aromatherapist for over two decades. She is the author of five best-selling books on aromatherapy and co-author of two more. She was a member of the working parties which set up the International Federation of Aromatherapists and the Aromatherapy Organisations Council. She is also a founder member and Fellow of the International Society of Professional Aromatherapists. She is the founder of Shirley Price Aromatherapy, the largest specialist aromatherapy training school in the world.

Shirley Price is the originator of a unique range of specialist skin care products and a supplier of top quality, genuine oils. She gives regular press, TV and radio interviews and contributes to specialist journals and magazines; she also lectures and teaches in many countries, and together with her daughter has produced a best-selling video on the subject of aromatherapy.

If UK readers would like to order any other Shirley Price books:

Aromatherapy for Babies and Children	0 7225 3107 9	£8.99
Practical Aromatherapy	0 7225 3906 1	£6.99
Aromatherapy and Your Emotions	0 7225 3862 6	£8.99

Please call our 24 hour mail order service: 0870 900 2050
(£1 per book will be charged for postage and packing)

For the best in health, mind, body and spirit books visit Thorsons .com

The Aromatherapy Workbook

Understanding Essential Oils from Plant to User

SHIRLEY PRICE

Thorsons

Thorsons
An Imprint of HarperCollins*Publishers*
77–85 Fulham Palace Road,
Hammersmith, London W6 8JB

The Thorsons website address is:
www.thorsons.com

First published 1993
This edition was fully revised and updated in 2000

20 19 18 17 16 15 14

A catalogue record for this book
is available from the British Library

ISBN 0 7225 2645 8

Printed and bound in Great Britain by
Martins the Printers Limited,
Berwick upon Tweed

Contents

'Fragrant oil brings joy to the heart
and a friend's support is as pleasant as perfume.'

Proverbs 27 v.9

Acknowledgements

I would like to thank Len, my husband, for his love, understanding and help while this was being written. My thanks also go to our daughter Penny, son Matthew and my long-suffering and efficient secretary Justine Finney. Valuable help was also given by my friends David Witty, Dietrich Wabner, Sjoerd Wartena and Trevor Leigh.

Introduction

To write a 'complete' book on aromatherapy is an almost impossible task. Not only would it need to be several volumes thick in order to cover every essential oil in use, but as new facts are being discovered continuously, a new edition would be necessary every year.

My aim, therefore, is to write about as many facets of aromatherapy as possible, while still maintaining a simple easy-to-read style. At the end of the book there is space for you to make your own notes and observations.

Since writing my first book on aromatherapy in 1982, the interest and enthusiasm of both my husband Len and myself has increased at least three hundredfold in one way or another.

A few years ago, we were becoming increasingly aware of the difficulty of obtaining essential oils of therapeutic quality from British suppliers, whose main concern is the much larger perfume and food industry market. Their requirements are different from those of aromatherapy and not so stringent as far as the wholeness of a natural oil is concerned. We therefore decided to attend an essential oil exhibition in France, which was solely for those requiring essential oils for health reasons, and as such, interested Len and myself very much indeed. It was a small, but wonderful exhibition; Len attended one or two of the lectures while I was making contact with the suppliers.

Buying essential oils is very much a matter of trust and liking people, and we were fortunate enough to find there one supplier with whom we had an immediate empathy. He even invited us to his home to see the area and the plants from which would come the oils we would be buying.

We spent four wonderful days viewing the fields and meeting the farmers. Already I was feeling excited that at last we were going to be able to give our therapists, mail-order clients and retail customers genuine, untampered-with essential oils, specifically for promoting the health and vitality of the body, rather than those imported purely for use in perfumes and flavourings, most of which need to be standardized, or have synthetics added to them.

We were finding ourselves visiting France several times during a year, to order the oils we would need and to watch (even take part in) the planting, hoeing, harvesting and distilling of the plants themselves, so we bought an old farmhouse in the region! We take groups of aromatherapists and interested clients to a converted ex-monastery two miles from our farmhouse, from where, for a week, we visit the fields, discover the medicinal plants on a mountain walk and watch the distillation process – fascinating! We take them to noted restaurants in the area, to the local *caves* (the wine-tasting cellars) and to a well-known market, passing on the way fields of lavandin (the gloriously purple relative of the true lavender plant) and the incredibly striking fields of massive sunflowers, all with their bright yellow heads facing the morning sun. All this under an amazingly blue sky, with the green grass and cornfields (which contain a host of vermillion red poppies) backed by the awe-inspiring mountains – the whole scene, with its accompanying aromas, needs to be experienced to be fully appreciated.

Why am I telling you all this? Because I want you to get a feel for the plants which provide us with their miraculous quintessence, and to appreciate, as I do now, that essential oils are not just powerful liquids in little glass bottles, but are representative of the individual plants and families from which they come, giving us their vibrant energy to help us to improve the quality of our lives.

Neither let us forget that plants such as these have, since life began on this planet, provided us with 'medicines out of the earth' as it tells us in the Old Testament. The amazing energy which some of us, including myself, call God, certainly completed his work incredibly well: a few moments spent thinking of the wonders of Nature and the intricate workings of the human body (and its ability to heal itself under normal circumstances) should be enough to convince us of the Power surrounding us. Would that we were all able to respect what we were given, treat it with care and use Nature's gifts efficiently to maintain good health all our lives.

My hope is that this book will help people to respect essential oils and to use them with efficiency and love.

1 *Setting the Scene*

The Mists of Time

When researching the history of aromatherapy it is well to remember that the word itself was only brought into being in the early 20th century, and its strict meaning is a therapy using only the aromas (i.e. the essential oils) from plants, not the plants in their entirety (i.e. herbalism). Thus, much of the history connected with aromatherapy is in reality the history of the use of *whole* plants for medicinal use – essential oils, especially as we know them, came later. Indeed, there are cave paintings recognized as being many thousands of years old which may be interpreted as showing the general use of plants for medicinal purposes. Phytotherapy (meaning a therapy using plants) encompasses many different ways of doing this – from the use of the shoots as in gemmotherapy; parts, or the whole, of the adult plant as in herbal medicine, Bach Flower Remedies and homoeopathy to the use of aromatic plant extracts only, as in aromatherapy and its non-medicinal counterpart, perfumery.

The origins of aromatherapy are lost in the mists of time, long before records of any kind were kept, though it is believed that crude forms of distillation, which is the main method by which essential oils are obtained, were practised in Persia, Egypt and India thousands of years ago.

Aromatic extracts were, and still are, taken from plants in many different ways; expression, enfleurage, maceration, solvent extraction and the method *par excellence* for aromatherapy – distillation. Distillation was originally used mainly for the extraction of exotic flower waters, such as rose and orange flower; the amount of essential oil produced was hardly perceptible, as flowers contain very little essential oil.

No-one can say for sure whether the extraction and use of aromatic material began in India or Egypt – suffice it to say that in both these countries the use of plants was, for thousands of years, an important part of their culture.

The Indian Story

In India the use of plants and plant extracts as medicines has been continuous from at least 5,000 years ago up to the present day. Ayurvedic medicine, as it is called, is unique in this respect, and one of the oldest known books on plants, *Vedas*, is Indian. This book not only mentions many aromatic materials, such as sandalwood, ginger, myrrh, cinnamon and coriander but also indexes the various uses of these plants for religious and medicinal purposes. Ayurvedic medicine, however, remained mainly confined to the area where it developed until fairly recently.

The Influence of Egypt

More is known about the development of plant use in Egypt and the surrounding Mediterranean countries; in fact the Nile valley became know as the Cradle of Medicine and among the plants brought to this area were cedarwood, frankincense, myrrh and cinnamon.

In Egypt 5,000 years ago, perfumery was so closely linked with religion that each of the gods was allotted a particular fragrance, with which their statues were sometimes anointed. It was the priests who formulated the aromas and the Pharaohs of the time asked them for perfumes with which to anoint themselves in times of prayer, war and love.

The Egyptians mainly used fats or waxes to extract the fat- or wax-soluble molecules from the plant material, and jars containing these aromatic unguents feature on many of the paintings in the Egyptian tombs.

To prepare an essence from cedarwood for hygienic use, and also for embalming, wood was heated in a clay vessel and covered with a thick layer of wool. The wool gradually became saturated with cedarwood oil and condensed steam; it was then squeezed, and the two substances were left to separate out. Here we can see the crude beginnings of distillation.

The Egyptians used plants, aromatic resins and essential oils in the process of embalming (prevention of the rotting and decay of once living tissue). They successfully preserved animals as well as humans by this method and the priests forecasted (correctly, as it happened!) that these bodies would last for at least 3,000 years.

Egyptian knowledge with respect to antisepsis and hygiene, so effectively demonstrated by mummification, meant that their influence has been felt right up to this century. In ancient Egypt the architects were among the leading scientists and Imhotep (who lived around 2750 BC) helped to initiate Egyptian medicine. One town, designed by Akhnaton's architect, was built with large square spaces for the burning of herbs, to keep the air germ-free. In the hot climate and with a lack of proper sanitation, the use of aromatic substances made life more pleasant – and safer.

Egypt and India were not the only countries to develop the use of aromas for religion and medicine (each country adapting them for their own particular requirement); the Assyrians, Babylonians, Phoenicians, Jews, Chinese, Greeks, Romans and eventually the Christians all burnt resins in religious mystic and purification ceremonies.

Greece's Contribution

About four or five hundred years before Christ, doctors from Greece and Crete visited the 'Cradle of Medicine' and as a result a medical school was set up on the Greek island of Cos, subsequently famous through the presence of Hippocrates (460–370 BC), who later became known as the 'Father of Medicine'.

A Greek, Megallus, formulated a perfume called 'Megaleion' – well known throughout Greece, no doubt owing part of its success to the fact that it was also capable of healing wounds and reducing inflammation.

The Greeks made a vital contribution to the future study of plant medicine by classifying and indexing the knowledge they had gained from the Egyptians.

The Roman Contribution

Through the influence of both the Egyptians and the Greeks the Romans began to be more appreciative of perfumes and spices – in fact, the word 'perfume' comes from the Latin *per fumum*, meaning 'through the smoke' and refers to the burning of incense. The Bible cites many references to incense, together with the use of plant oils and ointments.

De Materia Medica, a renowned ancient book written by Dioscorides, a Roman who lived in the first century AD, listed in detail the properties of about 500 plants. This information proved to be so influential that the book was translated into several languages, including Persian, Hebrew and Arabic. Dioscorides also told how he had come across the story of the doctor whom tradition claimed had invented distillation. This doctor had apparently cooked some pears between two plates in the oven and when they cooled, had tasted the liquid formed on the underneath of the top plate. To his surprise, this both smelled and tasted of pears, and as a result, he began to try and obtain not only this delicious 'spirit' as he called it, but others, in greater quantity. (Unknown to Dioscorides, others had already tried: in 1975 Dr Rovesti, well known for his research with essential oils, found in a museum a terracotta still from the foothills of the Himalayas – now 3,000 years old.)

As the Roman Empire spread, so did the knowledge of the healing properties of plants. When the Roman soldiers went on their long journeys to conquer the world they collected seeds and plants, which ultimately reached Britain, among other countries, and eventually became naturalized. Among these were fennel, parsley, sage, rosemary and thyme.

Baghdad was for many years the chief centre for rose oil from Persia (obtained by solvent extraction), and Damascus boasted a perfume industry.

Incidentally, it is thought that the Arabs were the first to distil ethyl alcohol from fermented sugar, thus providing a second medium which could be used for solvent extraction. (Around the ninth century Ibn Chaldum, an Arabian historian, tells that rose water was exported from Arabia to India and China.[1])

Early Distillation

In AD 980 a man was born who was to be responsible for making a vast improvement to the simple distillation units then known. Born in Persia, Avicenna (translated from the Persian name Ibn Sina) improved the cooling system, making it much more efficient, enabling the vaporized plant molecules and steam to cool down more quickly.

Avicenna further contributed to the world of essential oils by writing *The Book of Healing* and also *The Canon of Medicine*, used by many medical schools for centuries, and indeed right up to the middle of the 16th century, at Montpelier in the south of France.

Much more attention was now given to essential oils. Previously they had been regarded mainly as by-products of the much desired floral waters, as mentioned earlier. Other improvements to the distillation process followed (including refinements in the hardware used, due to the development of glass blowing in Greece and Venice) together with many new formulae for ointments and perfumes. One may almost say that the use of essential oils as we know them today began at this time.

During the Holy Wars, the Crusaders would have suffered the same stomach problems Europeans can suffer now in Middle Eastern countries. Without doubt they would have been given the same plant medicines used by the natives, including the floral waters and essential oils. On their way back, they would have stopped at various islands in the Mediterranean, where plant knowledge had been preserved from Roman times. From there they would have brought home with them perfumes and flower waters for their wives, relating stories of the successful Arab medicines. Thus the more advanced use of plants for medicines and perfumes became known once again in Italy and possible for the first time in the rest of Europe.

Development in the Middle Ages

During the Middle Ages the monasteries cultivated aromatic plants, some of which had been brought from Italy, such as thyme and melissa. In the 12th century a German Abbess, St Hildegard of Bingen, was known to have grown lavender for its therapeutic properties, using also its essential oil.[2] In the 14th century, frankincense and pine were burned in the streets, perfumed candles were burned indoors and garlands of aromatic herbs, spices and resins were worn round the neck to try to combat the deadly plague (Black Death), which raged throughout Europe during this time.

At the end of the 15th century (1493) in a town now part of Switzerland, Paracelsus was born, destined to become a famous physician and alchemist. He wrote the *Great Surgery Book* in 1576 and established that the main role of alchemy (the old name for chemistry) was not to turn base metals into gold but to develop medicines, in particular the extracts from healing plants (which he named the 'quinta essentia'). He felt that distillation released the most highly desirable part of the plant and mainly because of his ideas, oils of cedarwood, cinnamon, frankincense, myrrh, rose, rosemary and sage were well known to pharmacists by the year 1600.

As the gateway to trade with the Arabs was Venice, it was here that perfumed leather for gloves was first known. From here, Catherine de Medici took her perfumer with her to France in 1533. About this time, commercial production of essential oils and perfume compounds began in Grasse (perhaps due to her influence) and the area soon became established as the main perfume producing area, growing such plants as tuberose, acacia, violets, lavender and roses.

During the Renaissance period essential oils were much more widely used (the result of improved methods of distillation and the steady progress of chemistry) and around 1600, essential oils of lavender and juniper were first mentioned in an official pharmacopoeia in Germany.

The first botanical gardens were introduced into Europe before the birth of Christ and were later to be found in many monasteries. Because mainly medicinal plants were grown, botany became part of the study of medicine and under the influence of the Renaissance, universities teaching medicine began to have botanical gardens (known as 'physic' gardens). The first one of these was founded in Italy halfway through the 16th century, Britain's first being established in Oxford in 1621.

Aromatic Waters

Sometime during the 16th century Royal Hungarian Water was produced by distilling alcohol with fresh rosemary blossoms.

A French friend of mine, Claudine Luu, well known in France for her lectures and courses on essential oils (and her products) sourced the original recipe for this. The proportions are not given, but the other plant distillates in it were sage, rose and lavender.

Carmelite water (*eau des Carmes*) was produced by French Carmelite nuns in 1611 using melissa, which, like orange blossoms and rose petals, produces very little essential oil but yields delightfully aromatic water. Melissa water was popular for centuries and was never synthesized as are rose and orange flower waters nowadays.

Another famous water, which is still very popular, was introduced by a one-time Franciscan monk who left Italy to live in Cologne in 1665. His recipe for 'Aqua Mirabilis' (wonderful water) was brought to world fame by his nephew, J. M. Farina, and is known nowadays as 'Eau de Cologne'. Containing essential oils of bergamot, orange and lemon as well as lavender, rosemary, thyme and neroli (diluted in strong ethyl alcohol) it was used as a health-promoting lotion.

Progress in Britain

In 1653, Nicholas Culpeper wrote his famous herbal, from which people still quote today. Salmon followed with his *Dispensatory* (a pharmacopoeia) in 1696 and his *Herbal* (1710). By 1700 essential oils were widely used in mainstream medicine until the science of chemistry allowed the synthesis of materials in the laboratory. Around this time, during and after the Bubonic Plague, doctors were rather bizarre looking figures, walking through the streets wearing hats with large 'beaks', in which were placed aromatic herbs, so that the air breathed in passed through them and was rendered antiseptic. They waved in front of them a long cane with a big openwork top, which was also filled with aromatic herbs; this disinfected the air in front of them for double security!

The industrial revolution was in part to blame for the decline of the use of herbs in Britain. As people moved from the country to seek more profitable work in the new industrial towns, they came to live in terraced houses with little or no gardens. This resulted in a decline in the use of fresh herbs for cooking and future generations lost the art of incorporating them in recipes. Other European countries, less affected by the mushrooming of factories, continued to use them in the preparation of meals and also as remedies.

Scientific Development

By 1896 chemical science was becoming increasingly important. It was thought better to isolate the active therapeutic properties from plants and use them alone, or better still, to synthesize them – a much cheaper exercise, enabling large quantities of a uniform standard to be available (not possible with natural extracts alone). The drugs produced have proved to be very powerful and have an important role to play in modern medicine. However, synthetic copies of nature's healing materials tend to be toxic and do not appear to have the same respect for living human tissues. They tend to produce numerous side effects (some serious) which then need treatment themselves and a vicious circle is begun. Many of the people in hospital nowadays are there not because of their original illness but because of problems caused by the side effects of the drugs taken (iatrogenic disease). The use of natural materials such as herbs and essential oils does not give rise to ever-increasing dosage, as is the case with synthetics, to which germs may often become resistant.

Enter Aromatherapy!

The early years of this century saw a renewal of interest in natural methods of healing, no doubt stimulated by the unfortunate side effects beginning to be shown after long-term use of drugs. A few scientists began seriously to investigate and research the healing properties of essential oils, Rene Maurice Gattefossé being the most well remembered, probably because it was he who coined the word 'aromatherapy'. He had been introduced to the use of essential oils by Dr Chabenes, another Frenchman, who had written a book in 1838 on the enormous possibilities of utilizing aromatic material. Gattefossé (and others) used essential oils on the wounds of those who suffered in the terrible trench warfare of 1914–1918. In his research he discovered that essential oils take from 30 minutes to 12 hours to be absorbed totally by the body after rubbing on the skin. (This has since been corroborated by other researchers e.g. Schilcher.[3]) Gattefossé's book *Aromathérapie* was published first in 1937 and is now available in English.

Other pioneers worthy of note are two Italian doctors, Gatti and Cajola, and later Paolo Rovesti, who researched the psychosomatic effects of essential oils.

The use of essential oils under the name 'aromatherapy' reached Britain in the late 1950s, after an Austrian, Marguerite Maury, married to a French doctor and homoeopath, became intensely interested in essential oils, both working with them medically and researching their ability to penetrate the skin and to maintain youth. Aromatherapy was not introduced via the medical profession, but via beauty therapists, qualified in massage techniques, which is why, for so many years, aromatherapy has appeared to be 'a massage using essential oils'. As beauty therapists are not allowed in their code of ethics to 'treat' any medical condition, the main application of aromatherapy in Britain was to relieve stress and skin conditions by massage, and only massage. Partly because of this, and partly because much of the information on essential oils was tied up with their use in perfumes, the aromatic compounds called absolutes and resins were introduced alongside essential oils in treatment blends when aromatherapy with massage first appeared on the scene.

Through her lectures, Mme Maury was able to bring her ideas to beauty therapists in England, where she opened a clinic for facial and skin care treatments.

The beauty therapists were not taught how to select essential oils for each individual – selection was a closely guarded secret, for commercial reasons, and all oils used and sold on courses were ready mixed and blended in a vegetable carrier oil. All the courses I attended were like this and, being of an inquiring mind, I began to research the effects of individual oils, using my friends as guinea-pigs. The results spurred me on to prepare a course to teach aromatherapy in a more holistic fashion, teaching students not only to try and discover the cause of the symptoms shown, but to select essential oils individually for each client, and employ other methods of use. (At first I was criticized for giving away 'secrets' but soon all accredited courses will teach in this way.) Being already in the teaching profession was a great help, and gradually my classes expanded not only to include students from many different countries but also people from other disciplines, including physiotherapists, nurses, therapeutic massage practitioners and occasionally doctors. Aromatherapy is presently used in many hospitals and a number of beauty therapists now use the therapy in ways other than massage, which, after all, is how it should be!

The book of yet another Frenchman, Dr Valnet, made a great impact on the world of aromatherapy, especially after its translation into English some years ago. During all this time, aromatherapy was being used medically in France (notably by Belaiche, Girault and Pradal), essential oils being prescribed by doctors practising *'médecines douces'* (gentle, i.e. complementary, medicine – or parallel medicine as it is sometimes known there). Essential oils are stocked by pharmacies, though their purchase price, even when prescribed by a doctor, cannot be reclaimed through health insurance.

The technical book in French, *L'aromathérapie exactement*, by Pierre Franchomme, an aromatologist, in collaboration with Daniel Penoel, a medical doctor, contains some very valuable and interesting information on essential oils. In most French books the dilutions used are much stronger than a massage-trained aromatherapist would use, or indeed is taught to use. Somewhere along the line aromatherapy, as Gattefossé saw it, has acquired a slightly different interpretation.

Aromatherapy, as we now know it in Britain, has spread to many countries. Norway and Denmark were the first Scandinavian countries to enjoy the revival of essential oils and around the same time it began to develop in the United States and Canada; Australia, New Zealand, South Africa and Middle and Far Eastern countries following a little later. We have taught in most of these countries and the demand has necessitated us training teachers in many of them.

It seems right that a return should be made to natural remedies, which have been the mainstay of medicine for centuries. At the beginning of the 20th century, with no doubt the best of intentions, knowledge which had been painstakingly gathered together in many different lands was largely cast aside, and had it not been for the dedicated work and interest shown by a few people, mainly in France and Italy, this invaluable knowledge may have been lost forever.

Aromatherapy or Perfumery?

Plant aromas were extracted by solvent means long before distillation came into general use. The resultant compounds were not essential oils in the true meaning of the word, and were not used as medicines as were herbs. This is important, as there are many aromatherapists today who use absolutes and resins in their work; these are perfume and flavouring extracts and though, by inhalation, they can have an effect on the mind (as can any aroma, natural or synthetic), strictly speaking they are not for use in therapeutic aromatherapy. Nowhere in any French book on the subject are they included (except for benzoin) and as the man who coined the word aromatherapy always used the oils in a strictly medicinal way, i.e. in compresses, inhalations, baths, local applications in ointment form, intra-muscular injections and also internally – usually in honey water – this is no doubt the reason for their exclusion.

Some therapists use absolutes and resins (which contain a variable proportion of the solvents used to extract them – see chapter 2) possibly because when therapists began to select their own oils, these were available – and lent a rich aroma to a mix. At that time, none of us knew enough about the chemistry of such oils, nor about the copious adulteration of the exotic oils in particular (see chapter 2).

Research and Clinical Trials

Hundreds of thousands of pounds are spent on research, clinical trials and licensing for each allopathic or orthodox medicine, pill or potion which appears on the market. This is done with the best will in the world – to help alleviate suffering and disease. Unfortunately, medical science has only recently come to the conclusion that for all the care and time spent, these pills and potions often give side effects, sometimes even leading to death.

Although essential oils have not been clinically tested in this way (it would cost billions of pounds to test each oil and synergistic mix for each therapeutic effect of which it is capable) scientists feel that the same tests for proof of efficiency carried out on drugs should apply to essential oils. Drug companies are exceedingly rich and can afford to do costly clinical trials; users of essential oils have neither the money nor the facilities for such work. It seems to me unreasonable not to recognize traditional and repeated beneficial experiences over many centuries, simply due to lack of clinical trials – very important where the use of synthetic compounds of unknown potential is concerned (and also extracts from known poisonous plants such as the foxglove). Surely the same concerns are not as necessary for naturally occurring medicines which have been in use for thousands of years with extremely few recorded ill effects – nothing to compare with the number of adverse results from the use of drugs over barely one hundred years! Concerns over the use of essential oils are certainly not important enough to discourage their use and risk losing the natural heating agents given to us all. The proof of the pudding is in the eating, as we all know, and if essential oils had serious side effects they would certainly not have survived to the present day. People do not continue in the long term using remedies which do not work or make them ill.

God's world (a fantastic achievement) has existed hundreds of thousands of years already. Humans learned in their early days to use plants not only as food, but as medicines, long before modern civilization as we know it rocketed into being during the last three or four hundred years – particularly the last 100. How can we possibly think anything we have done in the last 100 years is 'proved' to be better? We are only just beginning to discover the harm we are doing to our own environment, to the atmosphere, even to our own bodies in this short time span – with such

things as car fumes, fast foods, steroids, synthetic vitamins and the unnecessarily bright and poisonous food colourings which the majority of
people consume each day.

I am not saying here that all plants are without risk, simply that the
clean record of traditional use together with up-to-date hospital research
projects, trials and general case studies should be sufficient. Misuse is a
different matter and is covered in chapter 6, as are the differences between
herbal medicine (in which many very toxic plants are used, e.g. boldo,
tansy, etc.) and aromatherapy (which does not use the oils from any of
these potentially dangerous plants).

Good, wholesome food is of itself a medicine, and it is a well-known
fact that the development of many diseases is in direct proportion to
the development of additives and synthetics together with the use of
growth hormones and fat inhibitors to produce bigger and better plant
and animal foods.

When looking back in history for the origins of aromatherapy, it is as
well to remember that aromatherapy has but a short history, the word
being coined only relatively recently. The history we have been looking at
has been that of plants, their extracts, compounds and essential oils.
Although the latter are the essentials of aromatherapy (in the therapeutic
sense), they are not limited to this particular aspect in their use, being
extensively used in the perfume, cosmetic, household and food industries.

'The Lord hath created medicines out of the earth and he that is
wise will not abhor them.'

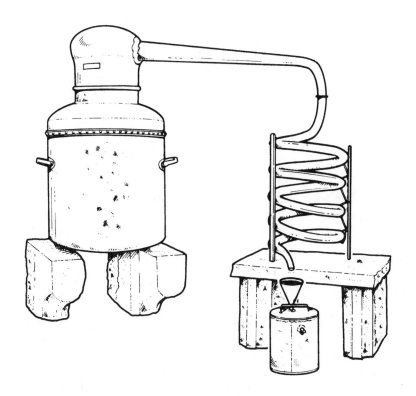

FIGURE 1.1: A 19th-century French lavender still (by courtesy of Raspail of Saillans)

2 Extraction Methods

Although the basic principles for extracting essential oils from plants remain the same as hundreds of years ago, tremendous advances have been made in the techniques used and the methods employed. Distillation is, and no doubt will continue to be, the most important of these.

Steam Distillation

Essential oils are contained in the glands, veins, sacs and glandular hairs of aromatic plants. Flowers, leaves and non-fibrous parts need little, if any, preparation prior to distillation. Tough stalks, woody parts, roots, seeds and fruits, however, need to be 'comminuted' (cut up, disintegrated or crushed – wood is grated) in order to rupture the cell walls, allowing the easy escape of the volatile oil. (Volatile is derived from the Latin *volare* – to fly.)

Distillation is still considered to be the most economical method of extracting essential oils from plant materials.[4] Some plants have to be distilled immediately they are harvested, for example melissa; if left even a few hours, the essential oil is lost – the yield from melissa is, in any case, very low. Some plants are left a few days, e.g. lavender, so that surplus water in the plant can dry out – this, by the way, slightly affects the yield. Some, like black pepper seeds, clary (clary sage) and peppermint, can be totally dried before distilling without losing any essential oil. It can be seen from these few examples that there is an art to distillation and that, especially for low-yield plants, much skill is needed. The role of the distiller is to achieve an oil as close as possible to the oil as it exists in the plant.

We distil water every day each time we boil a pan or kettle – the heat lifts molecules of water from the surface and they evaporate into the air, or condense as distilled water on the pan lid.

During distillation, only very tiny molecules can evaporate, so they are the only ones which leave the plant. These extremely small molecules make up an essential oil. Oils containing more of the smallest and therefore most volatile of these tiny molecules are termed 'top notes' in the perfumery world; those containing more of the heaviest and least volatile of the tiny molecules are called 'base notes'. Those in between are known as middle or sometimes 'heart' notes.

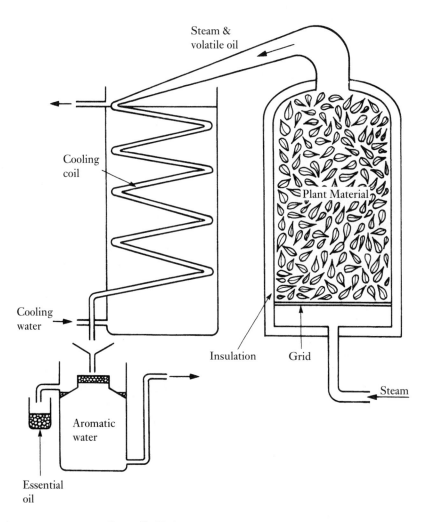

FIGURE 2.1: Steam distillation

When plants are heated by steam in a still (*alambic* in France), the essential oils present in the plant material are freed, evaporating into the steam. These tiny molecules are carried along a pipe together with the steam and as they get further away from the heat source they begin to cool. To hasten this process, the pipe passes through a large vat of cold water (the important addition to distillation contributed by Avicenna around AD 1000) and condenses back into liquid form. As the density of essential oil differs from that of water, it either floats on the top or sinks to the bottom (mostly the former), where it can be drawn off. The result is a pure, genuine, whole and natural essential oil – an aromatherapist's dream! This is the oil used in any reference or research carried out before the 19th century, when there were no synthetics to adulterate or 'ennoble' nature's gifts.

Distillation is more complex than I have made it sound (books have been written on this subject alone) but the underlying principle is simple to understand and remains unchanged.

Aromatic Waters

These are a by-product of distillation and contain some of the properties of the essential oil, even though it may be thought that because essential oils float on water they are not water-soluble. Some essential oil components do dissolve in water, and these, together with larger molecules from the plant (too large to vaporize, but soluble in water), form the aromatic water. Because of the presence of these other molecules, genuine waters have a different aroma from the essential oil of the same name.

The water from plants with a high yield of essential oil is normally discarded – directed into the nearby stream (large stills are always located beside a stream or river). However, with low-yield oils like melissa, rose and neroli, producers cannot afford to lose a single drop of the precious essential oil, so a special method called 'cohobation' is used, requiring a highly technical still and an experienced distiller. The basic process is as described above, except that, instead of using fresh water for each new plant load, the same water is piped back into the system, and used over and over again. Eventually, this water becomes saturated with the water-soluble elements from the plant (and water-soluble essential oil components). At this stage, every particle of volatile oil condenses and is collected at the end of the process to make a complete oil.

This saturated water is very concentrated and this strength is good for transport, as it saves on freight costs: it needs to be diluted with pure water to be comparable in strength with other plant waters. Lavender, clary and other waters from normal distillation are not as cheap as one would think (considering they are thrown away unless specifically ordered in advance), because of the cost of packaging and transport.

Before Avicenna's improvement to distillation and before cohobation was thought of, rose and neroli flowers were distilled simply for the water – the amount of essential oil obtained was negligible. In Tunisia, our friend Manoubi's mother, like many Arab women today, has her own tiny still, in which she makes orange flower water for her own medicinal and culinary use.

Unfortunately, unless one has a good connection in the country of origin (which, fortunately, we do), it is as difficult to buy untampered-with aromatic waters as it is to buy untampered-with essential oils (almost all rose water available in pharmacies is made with synthetic substitutes).

Aromatic waters can be made from plants which have no essential oil, by using diffusion.

Carbon Dioxide Extraction

This is a fairly new method of extracting essential oils, introduced at the beginning of the 1980s, utilizing compressed carbon dioxide. The technology calls for very expensive, complicated equipment (initially three or four million pounds' worth), which utilizes carbon dioxide at very high pressures and extremely low temperatures. With this method, more top notes (see above), fewer terpenes, a higher proportion of esters (see chapter 3), plus larger molecules, are obtained. The aroma of the resultant oil is more like the essential oil in the plant, as many terpenes in a distilled oil seem to form during the distillation process, which also breaks down some of the acetates (esters) in the plant material.

Carbon dioxide (CO_2) extracted essential oils are pure and stable and have no residue of CO_2 left in them. However, the therapeutic possibilities need to be verified for each oil on account of their different compositions and until there has been some research on this, it may be wise not to use them yet in aromatherapy.

At the moment the price is high; perhaps after a number of years, when the initial cost of the equipment has come down, the prices will be lower.

Hydro-Diffusion or Percolation

Percolation is even newer than CO_2 extraction and in 1991 we visited a unit in France. It was extremely interesting; most of the resultant oil had an aroma nearer to the plant than a distilled oil. The equipment, unlike that for CO_2 extraction, is very simple and the process quicker than distillation, the plant being in contact with the steam for a much shorter time.

This process works like a coffee percolator. The steam passes through the plant material from top to bottom of the container, which has a grid to hold the plant material. The oil and condensed steam is collected in a vessel in the same way as distillation. The colour of oils I have seen is much richer than that of distilled oils and time and tests alone will, as with the CO_2 method, reveal their true value in aromatherapy – it is certainly exciting! Percolation is not suitable for all oils; there are still a few practical difficulties to overcome (sometimes an emulsion is produced), but I am tempted to do a research project on one or two myself!

Expression

This method of extraction is used exclusively with citrus fruits, where the essential oil, located in little sacs just under the surface of the rind, simply needs to be pressed out. You can do this for yourself on a small scale: squeeze a succulent section of orange peel within an inch of a candle flame or lighted match and the tiny droplets of essential oil will ignite like baby fireworks. This shows not only the volatility of essential oils, but also that one needs to keep them away from a naked flame, as they are highly inflammable.

Expression is usually carried out by a factory producing fruit juice, thus maximizing the profit from the whole fruit. Most essential oil of orange comes from the USA, where millions of oranges are processed for their juice. The best essential oil does not come from there, as in order to maximize the crop, the trees and fruit are sprayed with chemicals, and these toxins reach the essential oil glands. This would not be so important if citrus fruits were distilled, as most pesticides and fertilizers, being composed of larger molecules, do not come through in the distillation

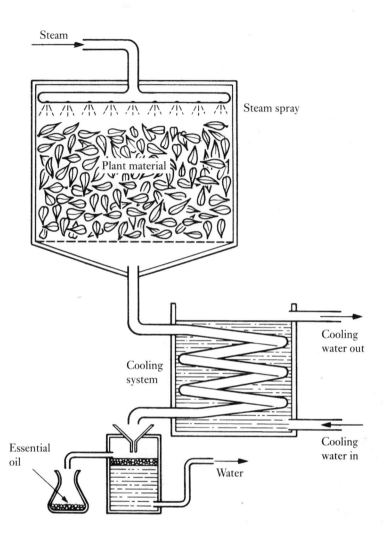

FIGURE 2.2: Hydrodiffusion

process. Nevertheless, as expressed oil is taken directly from the fresh peel without heat, it is best that citrus oils for therapeutic use be obtained from organically or naturally grown produce.

Cold-pressed citrus oils are special, in that they are acknowledged to be exactly the same composition as when in the plant itself. In many juice/essential oil factories the peel is steam distilled after expression, which releases even more oil (though of a poorer quality). Sadly for the aromatherapist, this is often added to the expressed essential oil to 'bulk' it, so care is needed when purchasing.

Although the oil was extracted by hand in the past (and collected in sponges), the size of the industry nowadays necessitates expression by machinery, when it is known as 'scarification'. In expression, both volatile and large molecules (such as waxes and other substances) are contained in the finished product, in contrast to distillation where only the tiny volatile molecules are collected.

The storage life of expressed oils is shorter than that of distilled oils, and although they have approximately 0.002 per cent antioxidant added to them, they are best kept in a cool, dark place (many people choose the refrigerator). In too cold an environment the dissolved waxes are precipitated, making the oil cloudy; this does not affect the therapeutic qualities (the wax has no therapeutic effect) so should this happen, simply strain your oil if you prefer it clear – warming the oil will not work, as the waxes will not go back into solution.

Solvent Extraction

Absolutes and resinoids are obtained by solvent extraction and are not classed as essential oils. They are highly concentrated perfume materials, containing those plant molecules which are soluble in the solvents used to produce them.

Resinoids

Resins are the solid or semi-solid substances exuded from the bark of trees or bushes when wounded (cut, as in a rubber tree). The gum-like substance produced does not exist in the tree beforehand but is produced pathologically solely as a result of the incision (poor tree!), and hardens on exposure to air. Various solvents can be used to extract the aromatic molecules from the resin, the most frequently used being hydrocarbons (e.g.

benzene, hexane or alcohols – each extracting different molecules). The solvents are filtered off and afterwards removed by distillation to leave either resinoids (from hydrocarbon solvents) or absolute resins (from alcohol solvents).[5]

Concretes

The extraction of concretes is similar to that of resinoids (hydrocarbons are used as solvents). For concretes however, plant material (leaves, flowers, roots, etc.) is used instead of a resin – this is the main difference. Most concretes are solid, wax-like substances and are much used in food flavourings.

Absolutes

An absolute is prepared from a concrete, by adding an alcohol to extract the aromatic (alcohol-soluble) molecules. The alcohol is then evaporated off gently under vacuum, leaving the absolute, a thickish, coloured liquid. The total process is much more complicated than I have made it sound!

Absolutes and resins are much used in the perfumery world, and although they can be useful in some applications of aromatherapy, it must be appreciated that they always retain a small percentage of the solvents used in their production. Some solvents may cause a substance sensitivity (see chapter 6) on certain skins, depending on the quality and quantity of the retained solvent. Adulteration is also a factor in this respect. Jasmine absolute, a favourite aroma for many people and possibly the most important fragrance in the perfume industry (there is no essential oil of jasmine available), is extremely vulnerable to adulteration[6] and available at a wide range of prices – reflecting the quality.

Enfleurage

Pommades were obtained from the enfleurage process used long ago (replaced by concretes), when petals or leaves were laid on trays of animal fat for many days, being replaced regularly until the fat used as a solvent was saturated with the plant extracts.

Adulteration

The perfume industry is far and away the biggest user of essential oils, followed by the food industry. These industries have to obtain an oil having the same chemical formula (therefore giving the same aroma and flavour) time after time, year after year. It has always been accepted in perfume and flavouring trades that essential oils are standardized and not always 100 per cent true, nor are they always from a named botanical species – they have no need to be. They are being used not to influence the health of the body, but as fragrances or flavourings – a totally different kettle of fish! When aromatherapy arrived on the scene, it was an incredibly small part of an essential oil trader's business – litres instead of tonnes. The trader could not be expected to undertake the uneconomic supply of special non-standardized or untreated oils for such a small section of his business. This is largely true today and unfortunately there are still suppliers of essential oils to aromatherapists who get their oils from such sources.

It will help to illustrate why it is important for the perfume and flavour industries to alter the original, natural composition of an essential oil if I make a comparison with wine. It is well known that there are good and bad years for wine; the same vineyard making its wine from the same vines each year will produce differences in aroma and taste from year to year. Weather and environment play their part in producing these changes, as they do with essential oil plants, altering the chemical formula of the oil produced. Furthermore, the same plant grown in another part of the world will yield a different oil again. Thus, the perfumer making up a well-known fragrance from a recipe including essential oils experiences a difficulty. For him, essential oils must be standardized, otherwise the end product would neither have the expected aroma, nor be acceptable: it is a question of adjusting (adulterating) the essential oils to achieve a legitimate aim.

Terpenes, a dominant feature in most essential oils, are sometimes removed to concentrate the remaining, more desirable constituents. The resulting compounds are known as folded or terpeneless oils, the terpenes often being used to adulterate another oil (see below).

Essential oils are also adulterated for commercial reasons – perhaps in an unethical way when operating in the field of aromatherapy. Before we bought our essential oils direct from the growers we were often asked, when ordering, 'How much do you want to pay?' In those days we did not realize what a complex business it was to buy essential oils, but we knew enough not to like being asked how much we wanted to pay, rather than being told the straightforward cost of the genuine oil!

What is Adulteration?

Adulteration, cutting, standardization, stretching, ennobling, sophistication – call it what you will, these terms, together with rectification (see below) mean that an essential oil has been altered in some way since leaving the still. Some of these processes are simple; some are quite complex, requiring sophisticated equipment. All these terms apply when the producer (or an intermediate further down the supply line) adds something to his essential oil to 'stretch' or standardize it.

Adulteration of essential oils can be carried out in a number of ways. The adulterant used may be:

1. an alcohol (to the inexperienced, the aroma is not noticeably different from the pure oil).
2. an isolate obtained from other essential oils (e.g. lemon or orange terpenes, which are available in huge quantities at extremely low cost).
3. a different, cheaper essential oil (and the claim may still be made in this (and no. 2) that the product is still a natural essential oil!)
4. a synthetic product, such as DPG (dipropylene glycol, which is colourless and odourless and is commonly added to bulk up lavender oil) or PEA (phenyl ethyl alcohol, a natural constituent of rose otto, which may be used to augment that oil).
5. an alternative, cheaper oil, somewhat similar, and substituted in toto (lavandin is often sold under the name of lavender, thus quadrupling the traders' profit – see chapter 5).

These methods are more or less accepted in the world of perfumery; indeed, I have been told by some that an essential oil may be regarded as pure if the oil contains 51 per cent of the original material; it is a fact that an essential oil is occasionally referred to as 'the soup' by some perfumers. This, however, should not be tolerated in the world of therapeutics, where to have a true to its name, untampered-with essential oil is of paramount importance.

I quote from the *Haarmann & Reimer Book of Perfume*[7]

'... bad harvests, political conflicts, exhaustion of the soil or transportation difficulties are imponderables which *make it impossible for the perfumer to rely on Nature's raw materials.*

Against that background, synthetic fragrance substances appear as economically indispensable substitutes for Nature's originals.' [my italics]

Fractionation

Here, re-distillation is carried out at low pressure in order to isolate the various chemical constituents, resulting in a terpeneless or a folded oil.

1. Terpeneless Essential Oils
These are essential oils that are concentrated by removing the comparatively inodorous and therefore (to some!) 'valueless' terpenes. The terpenes limonene and alpha-pinene, for example, oxidize readily and this alters their composition, resulting in changes to the aroma and to the therapeutic effects. This tendency of some constituents to oxidize makes storage of certain oils rather difficult. Also, having only slight solubility in alcohol, they give a cloudy appearance to the end product – a drawback to the perfumer and flavourist. De-terpenated essential oils are therefore 'more soluble, more stable and much stronger in odour'.[8a]

Terpeneless oils are not recommended for use in aromatherapy, because not only is the wholeness (and therefore the natural synergy) of the oil destroyed, but it now contains a higher percentage of the other chemical components; some of these may be the more powerful ones with which an aromatherapist has to take care even when present in lesser quantities in a whole oil!

Terpenes are removed by distilling under reduced pressure; as these are the smallest molecules present in essential oils they are the first to evaporate, eventually leaving the terpene-free oil in the distilling flask.

2. Folded Essential Oils
These are concentrated oils, differing from terpeneless oils in that they still contain varying amounts of terpenes. The process is halted wherever the perfumer wishes, with varying, known, percentages of terpenes being removed. The oils are referred to as singlefold, twofold – up to fivefold (where the greatest percentage of terpenes have been removed).[8b]

Essential oils are fractionated to remove other constituents too, e.g. bergapten (or bergaptene) which is a furocoumarin, not a terpene (see chapter 3). Fractionated oils are of use only in perfumery and the food industry, although some aromatherapists use bergapten-free bergamot oil because bergapten is the chemical responsible for photo-sensitization (yet use in sunlight is its **only** contra-indication! – see chapter 6). In my opinion this goes against the basic belief in aromatherapy that the whole, natural, synergistic mix of components, as extracted from the plant, should be used for maximum therapeutic benefit.

Rectification

Rectification ('putting right', or 'cleaning up') is carried out by re-distilling an essential oil which either has been contaminated with undesirable plant products (such as plant dust) through careless distillation procedure, or contains colour or aroma molecules undesirable for the perfumer. The end product is not necessarily an improvement in quality[8c] but is what the perfumer wants.

Synthetic Oils

Apart from adding synthetic components to an essential oil, a chemist can put together only synthetic molecules, to simulate the aroma of an essential oil, and, whatever plant name may be bestowed upon them, many cheap perfumes (and 'aromatherapy' toiletries) are totally synthetic (as indeed are many flavourings). It would be wrong of me to say that these have no effect whatsoever, as any smell, from whatever source, has an effect on the mind – even a bad smell – and can make one feel relaxed, awake, hungry or nauseous (for example, new-mown grass, frying bacon, nail polish remover, etc.)

However, a synthetic smell cannot, in my opinion, help a health problem without leading to side effects, as is often the case with synthetic drugs. There are scientists today who would argue with this and I believe such people are forgetting certain principles.

When science removes the therapeutic molecules or components from plants or essential oils, the administered result seems to give side effects. It is now appreciated that in the whole plant, or whole essential oil, there are many apparently useless components, including several that we cannot identify. These are believed to be 'quenchers' of the side effects which therapeutic agents in isolation could, and indeed do, cause. A good example of this is cinnamon bark oil. Cinnamic aldehyde, a major constituent of this oil, was found to be a severe irritant and the oil was therefore branded as an irritant. However, the complete oil, when tested, was found to be an irritant only on certain people – and to a much lesser degree.[9] The other components or constituents of the whole oil were quenching the irritant quality of the aldehyde, no-one knowing exactly which ones or how. (The whole oil may, however, be a *sensitizer* for some people – see chapters 3 and 6.)

If an essential oil can be made using synthetic versions of the chemicals that are known to occur naturally in the plant, the unidentifiable ones will be absent, therefore the result will not be a complete and whole essential oil. Thus it will most likely produce side-effects, as do other unnatural drugs. **Nature always knows best!**

There are scientists who believe that essential oils made in the laboratory will have exactly the same therapeutic effect as those made by Mother Nature; it is true that tea tree, the simplest essential oil, can be made in a laboratory and may help a health problem (though perhaps producing side effects with prolonged use). If asked whether there is any difference between synthetic and distilled tea tree, the scientist is bound to admit that there is a slight measurable difference in the carbon atoms, therefore giving a clue as to whether the oil is synthetic or not. He will also tell us that despite this, the properties are exactly the same! With more complicated oils, there are many unidentified components present in very small quantities, which cannot be imitated; hence such an oil would not be 'whole' as we know the meaning of the word.

This brings us to the question of vital force in essential oils. Almost every aromatherapist believes in this subtle, invisible, intangible quality that is not susceptible to any scientific proof. 'Life force' is thought to be due to some indefinable process (perhaps comparable to photosynthesis) whereby some part of the electro-magnetic energy of the sun's rays is converted into an energy which is stored in the essential oil cells in the plant.

The scientific community will quote the dictionary definition of vital force; 'the force on which the phenomena of life in animals and plants depend – distinct from chemical and mechanical forces operating in them'. In other words, once a plant is harvested it is dead.

The only difference between a living human being and a body in the immediate moment of death is this 'vital' or 'life' force. At that particular moment, nothing else has changed. The spirit or soul is a different matter for consideration; many religions, including Christianity, believe this lives on. In my opinion, the spirit of a plant (its energy) 'lives on' in its synergy (it is no longer *living*) and it is this special and unique mix of natural chemicals – which no human has been able to put together – which gives an essential oil its subtle, invisible, intangible, vibrant quality.

Quality

I have to be honest and admit that synthetic and adulterated oils will 'work' to a certain extent (in the latter there could be a high percentage of the natural oil present). It is the quality which is different. Optimum quality is paramount not only in order to get the best results, but also to avoid the risk of possible harmful side effects. A bonus is that less essential oil is then needed in order to be effective, a fact often forgotten by people who buy oils on the false economy of price. Organic oils are best of all (see below).

Despite the fact that we obtain most oils direct from the farming community, tests are carried out to determine the levels of the constituent components, as these are not the same each year. Because of this, an oil may not have exactly the same aroma each time you buy it.

Gas–Liquid Chromatography

It is possible to 'read' the formula of an essential oil using various techniques, the most common being the gas-liquid chromatograph (GLC). In this apparatus a minute amount of essential oil is injected into a temperature controlled, extremely fine, coiled, tubular column. The time taken (called the retention time) for each component to emerge from the other end of the column is different, depending on the molecule size. The quantity released is recorded, showing a peak on the trace (proportional to the quantity). This is a comparative test, not an absolute one, the retention time of known constituents having already been determined, to aid in the analysis.

As every batch of oil will vary in its percentages of components, one reading of each oil is kept as a 'standard'. This standard can then be directly compared to that of another essential oil from the same plant.

This technique shows any added adulterant having a retention time not evident on the standard. However it is possible to adulterate an oil low in a certain constituent, simply by taking that constituent from another, usually cheaper, essential oil, to 'correct' its reading. Sometimes a synthetic replica of a component is used, and occasionally, where a high concentration of one ingredient is desired, the oil will have a percentage of its terpenes removed, as in peppermint oil (see chapter 4). Aromatherapists should be wary of such an oil as this 'concentrates' the active components. Alternatively an ingredient may be augmented, as in the case of eucalyptol added to eucalyptus oil.

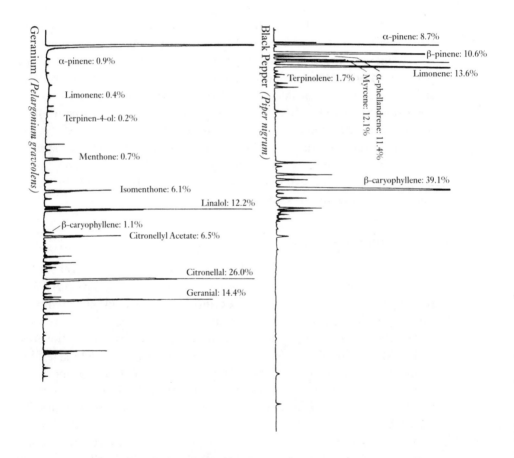

FIGURE 2.3: Gas-liquid chromatographs

Of all tests carried out on essential oils, the most common, apart from the GLC, are infra red, optical rotation, specific gravity, mass spectrometry (very expensive, but excellent) solubility in alcohols and ester content.

Organically Grown Oils

The term 'organic' has different meanings to different people. To the aromatherapist it probably conjures up a vision of aromatic and medicinal plants growing in unpolluted conditions. To the chemist, it simply means a substance which contains the carbon molecule, for example, sugar. The French term *biologique* or 'biological' is probably a safer term to use when referring to organic plant production.

Many of us would like to see a return to organic growing for everything – it is better for the soil, better for the environment and generally results in a superior product. However, organic growing methods entail heavy labour costs, sometimes yielding less attractive results – compared (sadly) with chemically assisted supermarket-type produce. The improvement in flavour of organic fruits and vegetables should make up for the – often – smaller size and sometimes less attractive appearance!

Often, produce claiming to be organic is not, and it is necessary for British produce to have a certificate, e.g. from the Soil Association, as proof, which can be asked for by any discerning or suspicious shopper.

The same principle applies to the growing and buying of organic essential oils, the certificates being awarded by the country in which the plants are grown, e.g. Natur et Progrès, Biofranc, etc. in France, Demeter in Germany, and so on.

It is obviously better for a plant to utilize the nitrogen, phosphorus and potassium (NPK) in the soil than to be fed with chemically produced NPK. The farmers in Egypt, where some of our oils come from, occasionally use potassium sulphate and ammonium sulphate from local natural deposits beside the lake. Pesticides are rarely, if ever, used, yet I must say that if a swarm of locusts set upon their fields, I for one would forgive them for using them – I would not expect them to sit back and watch their crops being eaten. After all, their livelihood is at stake!

I believe that to have organic plants for consumption, i.e. in the production of dried herbs and fresh fruits, is an admirable idea. Although we do stock certificated oils, we also have some which are not certificated but are from biologically grown plants; I am not keen to claim these as organic for the following reasons:

a) It is a very expensive process, involving inspectors examining the soil and testing the plants from time to time for fertilizers and pesticides. The certificate-awarding body claim money not only from the farmer, but also at each transaction through to the final one, so the price of the essential oil at the end is rather high. By the way, nitrogen, phosphorus and potassium do not come through in distillation.

b) It cannot be taken for granted that a field of biologically grown plants is always free from contamination. What about acid rain, air pollution, polluted ground water, aerial crop spraying, radioactivity e.g. Chernobyl, etc. – all beyond the control of the farmer?

Nevertheless, for those who (like several of our French farmer suppliers) believe in natural methods, the belief itself has to be the reason for wanting organic essential oils and if these beliefs are serious, it is a pity to have to escalate the price by buying proof, unless it is impossible to sell the crop (or the oils) without it. It may come to this one day, simply because some people will sell oils without certificates, claiming they are organic, when in fact they are not – just like the fruit and vegetable trade!

3 *Aromachemistry – the Chemistry of Essential Oils*

We are now going to take a look at the fundamentals of essential oils – the structure and effects of their chemical components. I want you to enjoy this chapter, and I hope you find it absorbing and stimulating.

Essential oils can be classified in several ways and if you know the chemical composition of an oil you can make a fairly good guess as to its therapeutic effects and possible hazards. There is no need for me to go into great detail – as my husband puts it, 'It is quite safe to drive a car without being a qualified mechanic, so long as we understand the simple basic principles of how the car works and we have learnt to control it.'

I shall explain only the basics, very simply and I hope clearly, so that you can appreciate the significance of the components which make up the oils – and their relationship with one another. This way, you will get to know these precious gifts of nature and be able to use them in an understanding and respectful way.

Everything in the world, both living and non-living, is made up of chemicals. Most of the chemistry I learned at school was about things that are non-living and have never lived – this is called 'inorganic' chemistry. The chemistry which includes all living things (and those which have once lived) is called '**organic**' chemistry or the chemistry of the carbon compound, since all organic substances contain carbon. The two main groups of chemicals in organic chemistry are referred to as chain or *aliphatic* and ring or *aromatic* (not necessarily meaning odorous).

Carbon, hydrogen, nitrogen and oxygen (this last accounts for nine-tenths of the human body!) are the basic building blocks of life itself, each of them being composed of atoms, the atom itself being thought at one time to be the smallest particle in existence.

Atoms

The building blocks of the universe! Every atom has a nucleus containing one or more protons, which are electrically positive, and one or more neutrons, which are neutral. Around the outside, depending on the particular atom, there are one or more electrons, each of which carries a negative electrical charge. These electrons are whizzing round and round the nucleus, rather like the earth orbits around the sun – ceaseless, never still. See Figure 3.1.

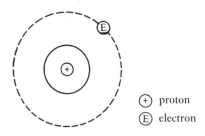

$\oplus$ proton
E electron

FIGURE 3.1: Hydrogen atom

The electrons orbit the nucleus at various distances from it. To feel really happy, the atom likes to have two electrons in the first 'orbit' (called a shell) around the nucleus – the second and further orbits or shells like to have eight.

As you can see from the diagram, a hydrogen atom is short of one electron – oxygen is short of two and carbon is short of no less than four! So each searches for and joins with other atoms capable of sharing electrons and therefore satisfactorily completing the number necessary for its stability. The atom is then content!

A simpler way to represent the 'discontented' or unstable atoms is to give them 'arms', i.e. – and =. These arms are called 'bonds' because they unite one atom to another.

Molecules

Once there are two or more atoms joined together, the group then becomes a molecule and Figure 3.2a shows a complete molecule of hydrogen, sharing the electrons.

You will notice that hydrogen only needs one more atom like itself to become stable. Oxygen, on the other hand, needs two hydrogen atoms to become a stable molecule of water (H_2O). See Figure 3.2b. If we give the carbon atom four hydrogen atoms it will become a stable molecule of methane, (CH_4) – Figure 3.2c, which is a gas; if we give the carbon atom two oxygen atoms (remember that oxygen has 2 arms) it will become a molecule of carbon dioxide (CO_2), also a gas – the one we breathe out (Figure 3.2d).

a)

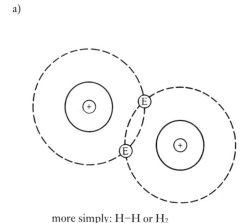

more simply: H−H or H_2

b)   H−O−H or H_2O c) $\overset{\displaystyle H}{\underset{\displaystyle H}{H-C-H}}$ or CH_4 d)   O=C=O or CO_2

FIGURE 3.2: a) hydrogen molecule; b) water molecule; c) methane molecule; d) carbon dioxide molecule

The bonds making up the water and the methane molecules are called 'single bonds', those making the carbon dioxide molecule are called 'double bonds', because there are two parallel bonds. Double bonds give a molecule a certain amount of rigidity, but they can separate fairly easily to provide an opportunity for other atoms to join in and share electrons as we shall see later on.

Now it begins to get interesting! Carbon atoms have a special ability to keep joining with other carbon atoms to form long straight or branched chains. Each time a carbon atom (with two hydrogen atoms) joins the chain, the molecule so formed is bigger and heavier than the one preceding it (see Figure 3.3).

We are nearly there!

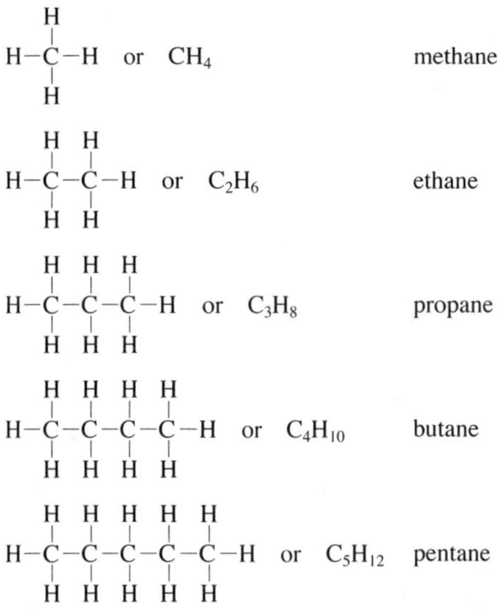

$$
\begin{array}{ll}
H-\overset{\displaystyle \overset{H}{|}}{\underset{\displaystyle \underset{H}{|}}{C}}-H \quad \text{or} \quad CH_4 & \text{methane}
\end{array}
$$

$$
H-\overset{\overset{H}{|}}{\underset{\underset{H}{|}}{C}}-\overset{\overset{H}{|}}{\underset{\underset{H}{|}}{C}}-H \quad \text{or} \quad C_2H_6 \qquad \text{ethane}
$$

$$
H-\overset{\overset{H}{|}}{\underset{\underset{H}{|}}{C}}-\overset{\overset{H}{|}}{\underset{\underset{H}{|}}{C}}-\overset{\overset{H}{|}}{\underset{\underset{H}{|}}{C}}-H \quad \text{or} \quad C_3H_8 \qquad \text{propane}
$$

$$
H-\overset{\overset{H}{|}}{\underset{\underset{H}{|}}{C}}-\overset{\overset{H}{|}}{\underset{\underset{H}{|}}{C}}-\overset{\overset{H}{|}}{\underset{\underset{H}{|}}{C}}-\overset{\overset{H}{|}}{\underset{\underset{H}{|}}{C}}-H \quad \text{or} \quad C_4H_{10} \qquad \text{butane}
$$

$$
H-\overset{\overset{H}{|}}{\underset{\underset{H}{|}}{C}}-\overset{\overset{H}{|}}{\underset{\underset{H}{|}}{C}}-\overset{\overset{H}{|}}{\underset{\underset{H}{|}}{C}}-\overset{\overset{H}{|}}{\underset{\underset{H}{|}}{C}}-\overset{\overset{H}{|}}{\underset{\underset{H}{|}}{C}}-H \quad \text{or} \quad C_5H_{12} \qquad \text{pentane}
$$

FIGURE 3.3: The chain increases by the addition of CH_2 each time

Isoprene Units

An isoprene unit is a molecule comprising five carbon atoms in a branched chain and is one of the two basic building blocks for essential oils. See Figure 3.4.

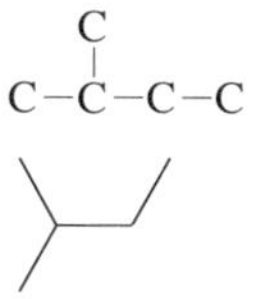

a branched chain, often denoted by
□
(hydrogen atoms omitted for simplicity)

FIGURE 3.4: Isoprene unit

Terpenes

Some terpenes are hydrocarbons, being made up solely of carbon and hydrogen atoms in a chain. Because they are in a chain they are termed aliphatic. Although they are not classed as aromatic, they do have some aroma, and play a part in the therapeutic effect of the whole oil. Perfumers are interested in the individual chemicals within an essential oil and sometimes those oils with a large percentage of terpenes are partially or completely de-terpenated – meaning that some or all of the terpenes are removed from the natural oil (an oil so treated is also known as a folded oil – see fractionation in chapter 2). As already explained earlier in the book, the big essential oil companies sell most of their oils to the perfume and food industries, whose requirements far outweigh those of aromatherapy suppliers. Unless the latter specifically state that they do not want a de-terpenated or folded oil, this is what they will probably be given, and where then is the synergy concept of a whole, natural essential oil for the aromatherapist?

Monoterpenes

Two isoprene units (ten carbon atoms) joined together head to tail, make what is known as a **monoterpene** (more often referred to simply as a terpene), which is a class of chemical compounds contained in essential oils. See Figure 3.5.

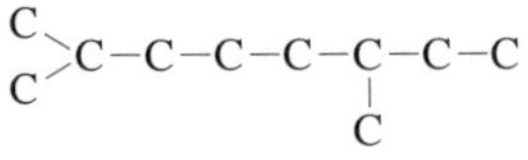

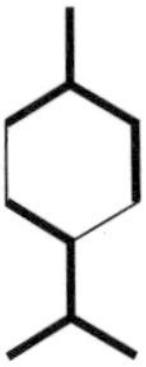

FIGURE 3.5: Cyclic monoterpene and chain monoterpene (each made up of two isoprene units)

Monoterpenes occur in practically all essential oils and their effects, although weak, are antiseptic in the air, bactericidal, stimulating, expectorant and slightly analgesic. Some are antiviral and others break down gall stones. As they may be slightly irritating to the skin, oils containing a high percentage of these should always be used in a carrier of some sort. All the citrus oils (except bergamot) contain a high proportion of terpenes, especially dextro-limonene (see Figure 3.6) and, although there has been one report of hypersensitivity to this material, it may generally be regarded as safe (allergic eczema involving orange peel has been attributed to limonene, but the case has not been proved). In fact, dextro-limonene is thought to be a quencher – i.e. it quenches any hazardous effects an oil may have. For example, when an oil containing a large percentage of dextro-limonene, e.g. mandarin, is added to lemongrass (a skin irritant, because of its high aldehyde content), the limonene in it quenches the irritant effect, rendering the lemongrass safe to use.[10]

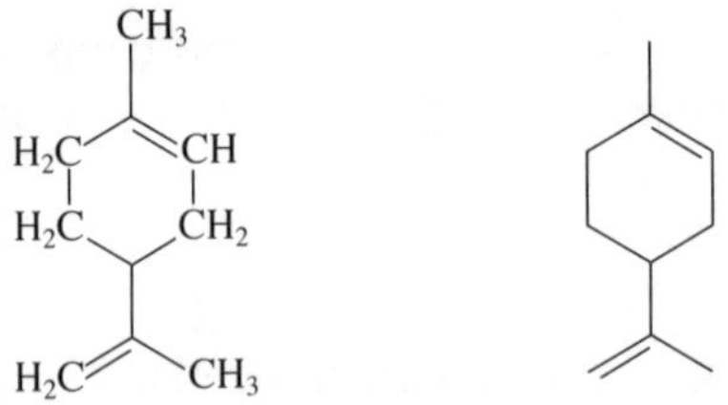

FIGURE 3.6: Limonene, a cyclic monoterpene

Sesquiterpenes

Now they start to look more complicated – don't worry! It is not necessary to learn these molecules – I show them only so that you can see how they get bigger and heavier, which explains why some are more volatile than others (see chapter 2).

If three isoprene units join together head to tail they make a longer and heavier chain molecule known as a **sesquiterpene** (15 carbon atoms), which is another class of chemical compounds. See Figure 3.7.

a)

b)

FIGURE 3.7:   a) Sesquicitronellene, a chain sesquiterpene
b) α-bisabolene, a monocyclic sesquiterpene

An enormous number of essential oils contain sesquiterpenes, such as bisabolene, found in black pepper and lemon oils. Another sesquiterpene worth remembering, because it occurs in practically all plants which belong to the labiate family, is beta-caryophellene. (Azulene is not a true sesquiterpene, though it often is shown as such and occurs in several oils – see chamomile, chapter 3.)

Sesquiterpenes are slightly antiseptic, bactericidal, slightly hypotensive, calming and anti-inflammatory; some are analgesic and/or spasmolytic (relieve muscle spasm or cramp).

Diterpenes

When four isoprene units join together this larger molecule is known as a **diterpene** (see Figure 3.8). There are not many essential oils with diterpenes as the complete molecule is rather heavy to come over in the distillation process.

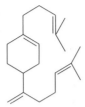

FIGURE 3.8: α–camphorene, a diterpene

Diterpenes are slightly bactericidal, expectorant and purgative, some are antifungal and antiviral and appear to have a balancing effect on the hormonal system.[11]

Now that we have an idea of what terpenes are, we can begin to look at them more closely.

The terpenes, of which there are many in nearly every oil, seem to be quite weak in their effects (though not insignificant). However, if the concept of a whole oil is to be recognized as important – which it is – they could well have a secondary use as diluents or quenchers to any possible side effect the oil may have if they were not there, as explained earlier.

Chain Building Blocks (Aliphatic)

Each of the terpene classes above (having 10, 15 and 20 carbon atoms respectively) may be regarded as 'chain skeletons', which can attract specific functional groups of atoms to form alcohols, aldehydes, ketones and (organic) acids, thus forming a myriad of different molecules, all having different shapes and therefore different therapeutic properties.

Ring Building Blocks (Aromatic)

These are the second building blocks for essential oils. Carbon atoms do not always join together in a straight or branched chain. Sometimes six of them will join together in a ring to form what is known as a benzene (or aromatic) ring. It is so called because the basic molecule formed is named benzene (and so many substances based on this molecule are aromatic). Nowadays it is more often called a phenyl ring, though all three names are used.

The shape formed by these six carbons may be regarded as a 'ring skeleton', and to it can be attached the same functional groups as can join a chain skeleton, to give yet another range of molecules – *phenols* (not alcohols this time), aldehydes, ketones and (organic) acids.

The phenyl ring can be represented diagrammatically in more than one way; these are easy to draw and to recognize, and using one of them saves writing out the whole formula (see Figure 3.9).

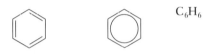

C_6H_6

FIGURE 3.9: Benzene ring or aromatic ring or phenyl ring

I show both diagrammatic forms for the sake of interest, but I recommend use of the second one as it is the most up to date and the least confusing.

A word of warning! When two isoprene units are joined together they may appear to be rather like the phenyl ring. However, if you look carefully, you will be able to see that the monoterpene has 10 carbon atoms, whereas the phenyl ring has only six. See Figure 3.10.

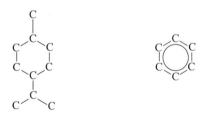

FIGURE 3.10: Monoterpene chain (10 carbons) and phenyl ring (6 carbons) [hydrogen atoms (H) omitted]

You may by now have a slight idea of the complexity and multiplicity of essential oil constituents, and I trust you also have a good basic understanding of the chemistry behind the formation of the two main 'skeletons' namely the aliphatic chain and the aromatic ring. These form the basis of all essential oils.

These skeletons are known as hydrocarbons because they are made up only of hydrogen and carbon atoms. Within the framework described there are many, many hydrocarbon relations, whose molecules are basically the same, but with slight variations. I will not confuse you by including all of these – you will meet their names in many aromatherapy books. *We* will concentrate only on the main ones!

The Addition of Oxygen

So far we have become familiar with two of the essential building blocks of life, namely carbon and hydrogen (forming hydrocarbons), and now we are going to introduce another element, oxygen. Oxygen is usually found as part of a functional group. There are many such groups, each altering the carbon chain or phenyl ring molecule to which it is attached, to form alcohols, aldehydes, ketones, etc. (as explained above).

Of the molecules we are going to look at, those having therapeutic effects – largely without toxicity – are alcohols and esters (which are interrelated with organic acids). Ketones, aldehydes and phenols, also effective therapeutically, need to be treated with respect as they are very powerful.

Let us take these molecules one at a time without worrying about remembering the *name* of each functional group – it is much more important to remember the 'family' name of the chemical formed by the addition of a functional group – alcohol, ketone, etc.

There are many different alcohols, aldehydes, (organic) acids, and so on in a single essential oil – essential oils are extremely complex mixes. In fact there is no direct, *simple* relationship between any one chemical constituent and the therapeutic qualities of a whole essential oil.[12]

Alcohols

The hydroxyl group (-OH) consists of one hydrogen atom and one oxygen atom; it is not very happy or stable as it has a free arm longing to link with another free arm. When this free *hydroxyl* group attaches itself to one of the carbons in an aliphatic terpene chain (by displacing one of the hydrogens) it forms an alcohol. Thus a range of alcohols may be formed (none of these is the same as that which occurs in wine and spirits! That is ethyl alcohol, which does not occur in essential oils).

Monoterpenols

When the terpene to which the hydroxyl group attaches itself is a monoterpene, the resulting alcohol is called a monoterpenol and these, like all alcohols, are comparatively easy to recognize as they all end in 'ol', for example terpineol, geraniol, linalool (sometimes spelt 'linalol') and menthol. They are strong bactericides, anti-infectious, antiviral, stimulating, warming, good general tonics and seen to be free of any hazard, including skin irritation. Because of this, essential oils containing a high percentage of alcohols may generally be regarded as good oils to use on children and the elderly. See Figure 3.11.

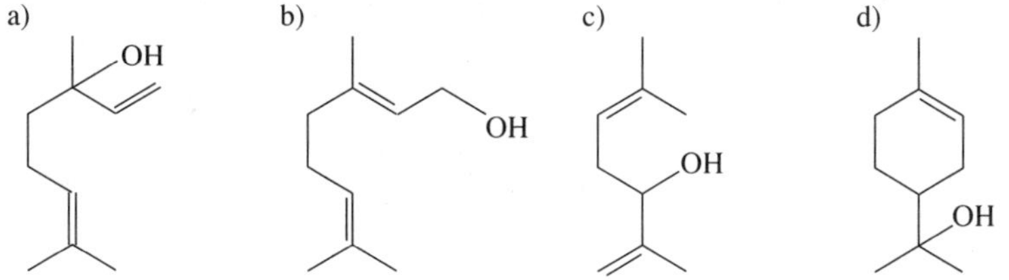

FIGURE 3.11: a) Linalool; b) α-geraniol; c) lavandulol, a chain monoterpene; d) α-terpineol, a cyclic monoterpenol

Sesquiterpenols

Should the free –OH group attach itself to a sesquiterpene molecule, it becomes an alcohol called a sesquiterpenol (see Figure 3.12). These are decongestant to the circulatory system, tonic and, like the monoterpenols, also non–irritating. Some have specific actions such as being stimulating to the heart or regenerating to the liver.

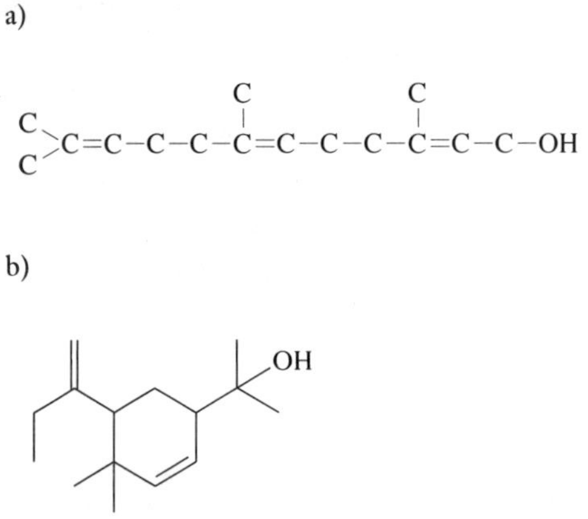

a)

b)

FIGURE 3.12:   a) farnesol, a chain sesquiterpenol; b) elemol, a monocyclic sesquiterpenol

Diterpenols

These are formed in the same way, by a free –OH group attaching itself to a diterpene molecule. Being heavier, they are not very volatile, so not many of them vaporize and come through the distillation process into the essential oil. However, they are very important, as their structure is somewhat similar to that of human hormones (steroid) and they appear to have a balancing effect on the hormonal system.[11] Sclareol (just small enough to vaporize) is a diterpenic alcohol found in clary essential oil and is claimed to be a hormone balancer. See Figure 3.13.

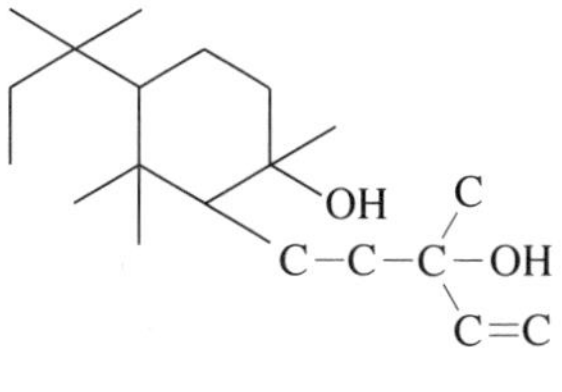

FIGURE 3.13: Sclareol, a diterpenol

So far we have seen the results of attaching the –OH group to molecules made up of hydrocarbon chains of various lengths. Now let us see what happens when this same –OH group joins a hydrocarbon phenyl ring.

Phenols

When the –OH group attaches itself to a carbon in the phenyl ring, the new molecule is known as a phenol, not an alcohol. See Figure 3.14. Phenols are very active and even stronger in their action than alcohols. Unfortunately for ease of recognition, phenols also end in '-ol', so it is necessary to learn the major ones. These include carvacrol, eugenol, thymol – there are many; some are present as phenolic ethers which can be neurotoxic. The latter mostly end in 'ole', e.g. trans- and cis-anethole – trans-anethole is less toxic than cis-anethole.[10] These are slightly more complicated and we will not go into their chemistry now. N.B. An exception to the 'ole' ending is the phenolic ether asarone, in carrot oil.

Powerful antiseptics and bactericides, phenols are stimulant both to the nervous and the immune systems *but* if present in significant amounts, the oil containing that particular phenol should be used with discretion, in low concentrations and for short periods of time. Phenols can be skin irritants if used incorrectly.

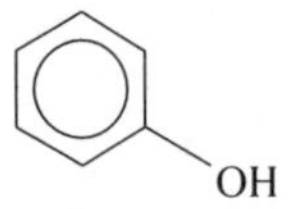

FIGURE 3.14: Phenol

Aldehydes

To make an aldehyde, both the carbonyl group (=O) and a hydrogen atom (-H) attach themselves to a carbon atom in either a chain or a ring molecule. See Figure 3.15.

Aldehydes are very important to the perfumer because they very often have a powerful aroma. There is no mistaking an aldehyde as they are referred to by the use of that word, or their names end in 'al'.

The properties of aldehydes fall somewhere between alcohols and ketones though they are not such consistent and anti-infectious agents as alcohols and tend to be skin irritants to some degree (see chapter 6).

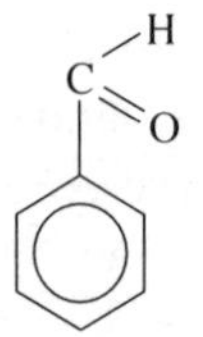

FIGURE 3.15: Benzaldehyde

A few aldehydes are skin sensitizers, which means they may, on certain people, cause a reaction such as a skin rash, which may appear whenever the same aldehyde is met with in any other oil.

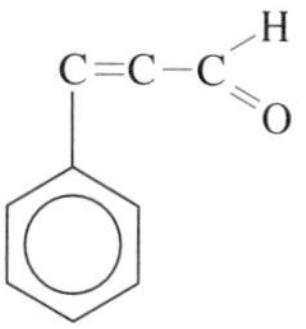

FIGURE 3.16: Cinnamic aldehyde

Cinnamic aldehyde (Figure 3.16), when isolated from cinnamon bark oil, can be a skin sensitizer, but when the whole oil (diluted and tested on humans) is used, it has been found not to be so.[9] It should nevertheless be used with care, as on certain hyper-sensitive skins, unless well diluted, it can be a skin irritant. Citral, an aldehyde (consisting of geranial and neral) present in lemon oil (5 per cent), is a powerful irritant when isolated; in the whole oil its possible hazards are cancelled by the presence of the other 95 per cent of constituents, most of which are terpenes. Many of the known (and unknown) constituents of an oil act as 'quenchers' (i.e. they prevent side effects occurring). Mixing an oil containing citral with an oil containing an equal amount of dextro-limonene can negate its irritant properties altogether (see under monoterpenes earlier in this chapter).

Aldehydes are anti-inflammatory, anti-infectious, tonic, hypotensive, calming to the nervous system and generally temperature reducing.

If an oil containing aldehydes is stored for any length of time or in poor conditions, unwanted acids can form from the precious therapeutically active aldehydes, rendering the oil almost useless for aromatherapy purposes.

Ketones

We now meet the carbonyl group again, =O, which attaches itself to a carbon on either a chain or a ring molecule, creating a ketone (see Figure 3.17).

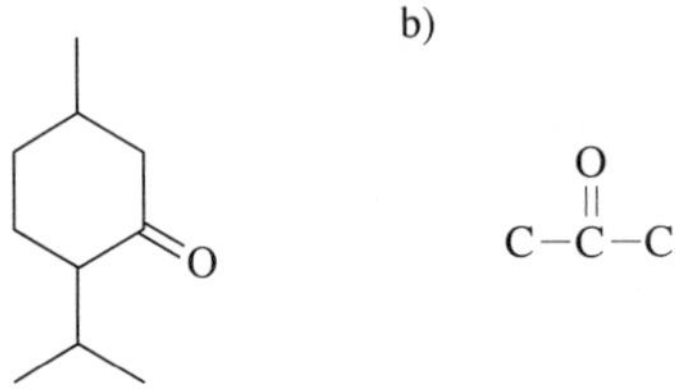

FIGURE 3.17: a) menthone; b) acetone (ketones)

These are easy to identify as they always end in 'one'. (N.B. A false friend is asarone, which is a phenolic ether in carrot oil.) A common one, not occurring in essential oils, but known to most people, is acetone (nail polish remover). Fortunately, ketones are not present in the majority of essential oils – I say 'fortunately' because many of them are not 'user friendly' and have to be employed with knowledge and care, as several are neurotoxic. There is no scientific proof that all ketones are hazardous and generally (and fortunately) those which are known to be very much so occur in oils not used by aromatherapists, e.g. tansy, buchu, thuja, rue, etc.

Oils used in aromatherapy which contain significant amounts of ketones are aniseed, caraway, hyssop, pennyroyal and sage, and in France, only pharmacists may sell hyssop and sage oils. It is thought that the ketone in hyssop (pinocamphone) may provoke an epileptic fit **in someone predisposed to them** and that a few ketones, e.g. thujone and pulegone, **if used in overdose**, may provoke a miscarriage.

At the EOTA conference (June 1990) at Brunel University, Dr K. Tyman said that 'there are 4 different thujones and a change in molecular shape means a change in effect'. Dr Tyman made what I feel to be a most important statement, which explains why sage, supposedly very hazardous because of its high thujone content, does not in practice appear to be so.

He explained that because the thujone molecule can arrange itself in four different ways (alpha-thujone, beta-thujone, etc.) it is feasible to expect all four to have different pharmacological effects; therefore it may be that not all thujone molecule shapes will necessarily present a hazard.

Carvone, for example, present in caraway and dill oils (the latter is an ingredient in gripe water for babies), is assumed to have the hazards of all ketones, yet there is no evidence to prove this. In fact, it is believed that some ketones (like carvone) may be completely harmless. There are two forms of carvone, laevo-carvone and dextro-carvone, which may, as with the thujones, have different pharmacological effects. The properties of the two forms of carvone are different and they certainly have different aromas. Having said that, until further information comes to light we should take care with all oils containing ketones in any appreciable amount, just to be on the safe side – and it pays to know your chemistry!

Provided caution is exercised and oils containing ketones are well diluted (1–2 per cent maximum) and not used too often or for too long, their effects are calming and sedative, they break down mucus and fat and encourage the healing of wounds by the formation of scar tissue. Certain ketones are digestive, others are analgesic, stimulant or expectorant.

Acids and Esters

Organic acids are nothing like *in*organic acids, which are potentially dangerous e.g. sulphuric acid.

Inorganic acid + alkali = inorganic salt + water

Organic acid + alcohol = ester + water

Acids and esters are based on the carboxyl group (see Figure 3.20b).

Acids in their free state are quite rare in essential oils and occur only in minute quantities. See Figure 3.18. As they have no known hazards there is no need to go into greater detail than to say they are anti-inflammatory. I mention them mainly so that you can follow the molecular progress to an ester.

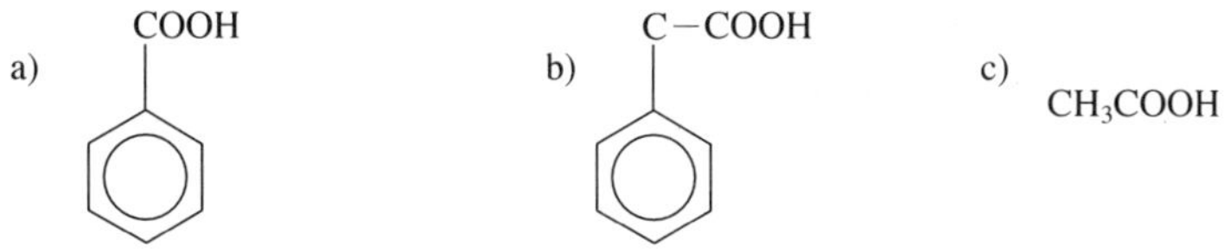

FIGURE 3.18: a) benzoic acid; b) phenylacetic acid (neroli); c) acetic acid (found in aromatic waters)

Acids are mostly found in essential oils in a combined state with esters, which we shall be looking at next.

There is no ester group as such (like the hydroxyl or carboxyl groups mentioned earlier) because an ester is the result of the reaction between an organic acid and an alcohol to give an ester plus water. See Figure 3.20a.

organic acid + alcohol ⟶ ester + water

FIGURE 3.19

The reverse can also happen; an acid plus alcohol is the result of the reaction between an ester and water. This is why I said above that acids are found 'in a combined state' in essential oils – it is possible that an interchange can be going on all the time. Perhaps this may be why esters are good balancers.

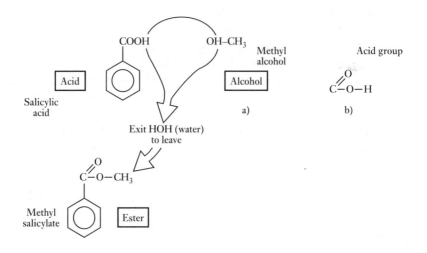

FIGURE 3.20: Formation of an ester

The last part of an ester's name is nearly always 'ate', making it another component easy to recognize (in some cases, the name ester is used).

Esters are gentle in action and are free from hazard except for methyl salicylate in wintergreen and birch oils (over 90 per cent), which are not recommended for use by aromatherapists. Esters generally are anti-inflammatory and are effective on skin rashes and other skin problems. They can both calm and uplift, combining the calming properties of ketones with the tonic virtues of alcohols, so they are very balancing, especially to the nervous system.

Oxides

These are rare in essential oils with the exception of 1,8-cineole, also known as eucalyptol. Some oxides have the name 'oxide' at the end, making recognition easier.

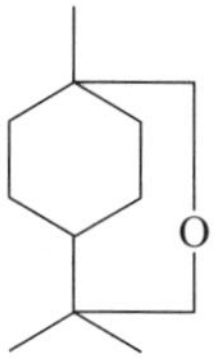

FIGURE 3.21: 1,8-cineole, an oxide

1,8-cineole (eucalyptol) – see Figure 3.21 – is found in a number of oils and its major effect is due to its mucolytic property, useful in coughs, colds and any congestion in the respiratory tract. It can be a skin irritant and in this respect any oil containing a two-figure percentage needs to be used with restraint.

This group tends to be confusing, and it seems uncertain whether some oxides are in fact phenols or phenolic ethers – even experts have differing opinions or are not sure themselves. To be safe, give them the same consideration and prudent use as recommended for the phenols. 1,8-cineole may also be described as a bicyclic ether.[13]

Lactones

Lactones are easy to remember because they occur mostly in expressed oils, being too large to come over in distillation. Jasmine absolute has been found to contain a lactone, but as you will remember, this oil is not an essential oil, as it is not obtained by distillation and therefore larger molecules can pass into the solvent used for the extraction process.

As the percentage of lactones present in any oil is extremely low, they may generally be regarded as non-toxic. They have been found to be more effective than ketones for lowering temperatures and relieving catarrh, and are the components responsible for skin photosensitization.

Lactones are widely distributed in nature; the most important members of this class (or chemical family) occurring in essential oils are the coumarins and coumarin derivatives.

Coumarins and Furocoumarins

Coumarins are generally found to be sedative and calming yet at the same time uplifting and refreshing. They are also noted for their anti-coagulating properties, which makes them good hypotensives. See Figure 3.22.

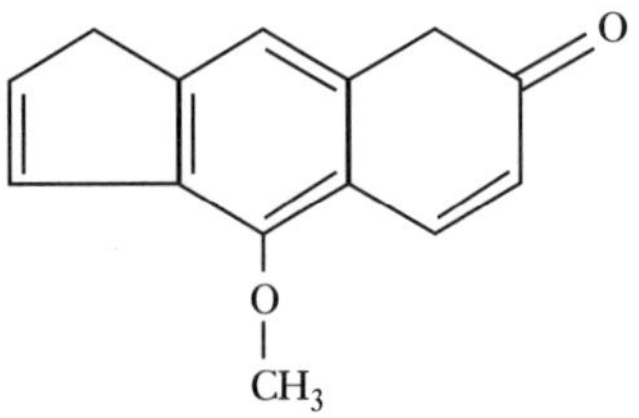

FIGURE 3.22: Bergaptene, a coumarin

Furocoumarins, closely related to coumarins, are noted for their hazards in connection with sunbathing. They are photosensitizers and should not be used immediately before going into the sun or onto a sunbed (see chapter 6). Bergaptene, found in bergamot oil (not a terpene and sometimes spelt without the final 'e'), is the best-known example.

Two hours after applying complete bergamot oil (see folded oils – chapter 2) suitably diluted in a carrier, there is no longer a great risk of adverse reactions due to the sun; by that time the oil is safely absorbed into the bloodstream.[14]

Ethers (Not to be confused with esters)

Here we have yet another component which occurs but rarely in essential oils and can be confusing. Like phenols and phenolic ethers, the properties of ethers are anti-depressant, anti-spasmodic and sedative.

Conclusion

An essential oil is always a complex cocktail of many different naturally occurring components; there are several different kinds of terpenes, alcohols, phenols, ketones, esters and so on in each oil, and these vary from harvest to harvest and plant to plant. The actions of any whole essential oil are difficult to forecast from this complicated make up; I repeat, there is no direct *simple* relationship between the chemical constituents and the therapeutic qualities (or even the hazards) of an essential oil.[12]

No one in the aromatherapy world understands or knows everything to do with essential oils, so take heart! There is also no way in which a book like this can cover each constituent known of every single oil, but simply by being acquainted with the main constituent families you may be able to see some sort of pattern emerging in relation to therapeutic effects.

There are, nevertheless, some essential oils whose chemical constituents do not seem to conform to their expected pattern and are the 'black' (or sometimes perhaps, the 'white'!) sheep of their family. There are also trace elements which show up on a gas-liquid chromatograph (see chapter 2), but have so far not been identified – these too must surely play an important part in the eventual effect of the final chemical 'cocktail'.

The above points (plus climate and soil variants) may help to explain why no document or book lists every minor chemical, or even gives the same proportions of the major ones. It would take years to research and would take up many volumes! (Guenther's well-respected reference work on essential oils comprises six thick volumes, without including any therapeutic effects!)

May I suggest that if you have found this chapter (so far) a bit difficult, yet you wish to understand it, you come back to it later. Read it again up to the isoprene unit, perhaps drawing the molecules as you go along, moving on to each new chemical family only when you fully understand how the previous one was formed.

Perhaps you already knew it all, or have neither the wish nor the need to pursue the intricacies of these simple to use and wonderful liquids!

In either case I hope you found it interesting.

Electrical Classification of Essential Oils

The therapeutic effects of the different chemicals we have been looking at can be shown by charting the reaction of essential oils and their components to electricity and water. There has been a lot of work done in France by Franchomme, based on investigations begun by Vincent and Mars, to determine the polarity of each chemical constituent in order to discover whether these follow an overall pattern. It presents a fascinating concept and has given very interesting results.[15]

When essential oil molecules are sprayed between two electric plates (one positively charged and one negatively charged) they will be attracted either to one plate or the other. This attraction stems from the chemical components, each of which has either a negative or a positive charge. Opposites attract, so negative components go towards the positive plate and vice versa. When a component from one chemical family is sprayed between the plates, it is attracted either to the negative or the positive plate. Aliphatic aldehydes (chain based), esters and ketones are attracted towards the negative plate; alcohols, aromatic aldehydes (ring based), monoterpenes, oxides, phenols and phenolic ethers towards the positive one; the sesquiterpenes, lactones and coumarins are neutral and are not attracted – some are slightly more negative – others more positive. See Figure 3.23.

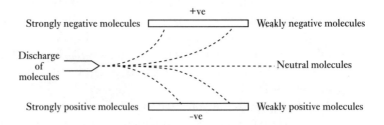

FIGURE 3.23: Movement of alcohol molecules

Essential oils are slightly soluble in water – this is due to the hydrophilic (soluble) or hydrophobic (insoluble) factor of each chemical family. Alcohols, all aldehydes, phenols, ketones, lactones and coumarins are soluble to some degree; monoterpenes and sesquiterpenes are insoluble, as are most of the esters; oxides and phenolic ethers fall in the middle, as do a relatively small proportion of the esters. See Figure 3.24.

With a four-way grid like this, it is easy to see which constituents from the essential oils are cooling and which are warming; which are calming and which are stimulating (Figure 3.25).

See how top and bottom, left and right, and opposite quadrants, complement each other; using a combination of these opposites, essential oils can be selected to treat the whole person. Franchomme's approach is that there is a relationship between the chemical components and the effects – if you know the chemical constituents it gives at least an idea of the effect of an essential oil containing these. I am told that he and his colleagues have carried out many clinical experiments in French hospitals to verify his work.

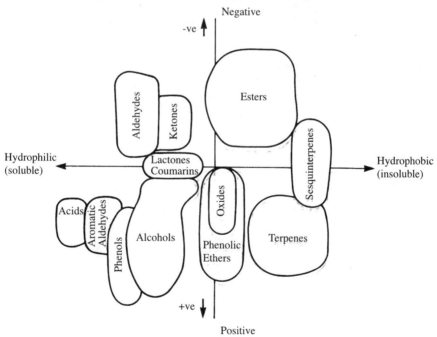

FIGURE 3.24: Polarity and solubility of individual components of essential oils (adapted from grid originated by Roger Jallois and published in *Aromathérapie Exactement*)

There is much work being done and more yet to be done on these fascinating creations of nature, essential oils. Even though I have only touched
the tip of the iceberg, I trust I have awakened in you a desire to utilize the
information in it to the good of your own health and, if you are an
aromatherapist, of that of your clients.

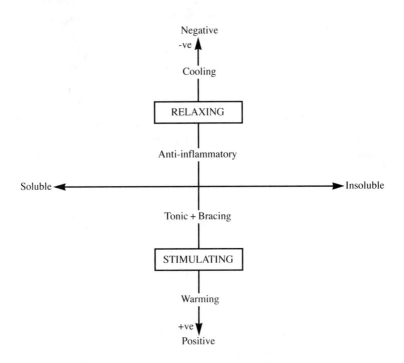

FIGURE 3.25: Basic effects of individual constituents

TABLE 1: Chemical Constituents of Essential Oils and their Effects

	Acids	Alcohols (mono)	Alcohols (sesqui)	Aldehydes	Coumarins	Esters	Ethers (phenolic)	Ketones	Lactones	Oxides	Phenols	Terpenes (mono)	Terpenes (sesqui)
Abortifacient								X					
Analgesic								X			X	X	X
Air Antiseptic												X	
Antiseptic				X							X	X	X
Anticoagulant					X			X					
Antifungal				X		X		X	X				
Anti-infectious		X	X	X			X				X		
Anti-inflammatory	X			X		X	X	X					X
Antispasmodic						X	X				X		X
Antiviral		X		X							X	X	
Bactericidal		X	X								X	X	X
Balancing						X							
Cicatrisant						X		X			X		
Decongestant, circulatory			X										
Digestive								X			X		
Diuretic											X		
Expectorant								X	X	X	X	X	
Hepatic		X	X										
Hypotensive			X	X	X								X
Immune System Balancer		X											
Immunostimulant											X		
Lipolytic								X					
Mucolytic								X	X	X	X		
Neurotoxic							X	X					
Phototoxic					X				X				
Relaxant				X	X	X	X	X					X
Sedative					X			X	X				
Skin Irritant				X							X	X	X
Skin Sensitizing				X					X				
Stimulant		X						X				X	
Temperature Reducing			X	X					X				
Tonic, nerve (uplifting)		X	X		X	X	X				X		
Tonic (general)		X	X	X									
Vasoconstrictive		X											

TABLE 2: Some Chief Chemical Constituents of Essential Oils

This table simply gives an idea of a few of the chemicals in selected essential oils and is not meant to be comprehensive.

Key
t = trace
s = small amount
m = medium amount
l = large amount

Column groups: columns *Bisabolol* through *Thujanol +* = **ALCOHOLS**; *Cinnamic Aldehyde* through *Neral* = **ALDEHYDES**; *Benzyl Acetate* through *Neryl Acetate* = **ESTERS**.

COMMON NAME (LATIN NAME)	Bisabolol	Borneol	Cedrol	Citronellol	Farnesol	Fenchol	Geraniol	Globulol	Linalol	Menthol	Nerol	Pinocarveol	Sabinol	Sclareol	Alpha-Terpineol	Terpinen-4-ol	Thujanol +	Cinnamic Aldehyde	Citral	Citronellal	Geranial	Neral	Benzyl Acetate	Bornyl Acetate	Citronellyl Acetate	Geranyl Acetate	Linalyl Acetate	Neryl Acetate
Basil, Exotic (*Ocimum basilicum v. basilicum*)		t				t			t							t												
Basil, European, sweet (*O. basilicum v. album*)				m					l																		(around 8%)	
Bergamot (*Citrus bergamia*)				s					l		s				s				l								m	
Black Pepper (*Piper nigrum*)									s				s		s													
Chamomile, German (*Chamomilla recutita*)	s		s														t											
Chamomile, Moroccan (*Ormenis mixta*)		(santalinol 30%)							t		s										t					s	t	s
Chamomile, Roman (*Anthemis nobilis*)	s		s										s														(around 60%)	
Clary (*Salvia sclarea*)									m					s													l	
Cypress (*Cupressus sempervirens*)			s										s															
Eucalyptus (*Eucalyptus globulus*)								s																				
Fennel (*Foeniculum vulgare*)						s																						
Frankincense (*Boswellia carteri*)	s		s																									
Geranium (*Pelargonium graveolens*)				m			m		t		t				t				t	t					s	s	s	
Grapefruit (*Citrus paradisi*)				s															s	s	s							
Hyssop (*Hyssopus officinalis*)	s						s		t																		t	t
Juniper (*Juniperus communis*)	s													s														
Lavandin (*Lavandula hybrida*)	s								m																	s	t	m
Lavender (*Lavandula angustifolia*)		t					t		l						t	s											t	l
Lemon (*Citrus limon*)							t		t						t	t			s	t	s	t				s	t	t
Lemongrass (*Cymbopogon citratus*)				t	t				t		t				t				l	t	s	s					m	m
Marjoram, Spanish (*Thymus mastichina*)	t						t		m			t			s	t	t											
Marjoram, sweet (*Origanum majorana*)									s			s			m	m	s	s								t	t	s
Melissa, True (*Melissa officinalis*)				s	s		s		s		s								m	s	m	s					s	s
Neroli (*Citrus aurantium amara*)		(nerolidol 6%)					s		m		s				s								t			s	l	s
Nutmeg (*Myristica fragrans*)	t						t	t								m												
Orange, sweet (*C. aurantium sinensis*)				t					t		t				t	t			t		t						t	t
Patchouli (*Pogostemon patchouli*)	(patchoulol 40%)																	t									(around 18%)	
Peppermint (*Mentha piperita*)										l																	(menthyl acetate 8%)	
Petitgrain (*Citrus aurantium amara*)				t			s		m		s				s											s	l	s
Pine (*Pinus sylvestris*)	s																							s				
Rose Otto (*Rosa centifolia*)				m	s		m		t		m										t						(around 5%)	
Rosemary (*Rosmarinus officinalis*)		m							s						s	s								s				
Sage (*Salvia officinalis*)	s								s						s	s	t							s			s	
Tea Tree (*Melaleuca alternifolia*)									t						s	l												
Thyme (*Thymus vulgaris* – phenols)	s																											
Thyme, sweet (*Thymus vulgaris* – alcohols)							l	or	l		——	or	——				m										s	s
Ylang ylang (*Cananga odorata*)					s		s		l												s		s				s	

Legend (left header block):

trace — t
small amount — s
medium amount — m
large amount — l

| | KETONES | | | | | | | OXIDES | PHENOLS | | | | | | | | TERPENES (MONO-) | | | | | | | SESQUI- | | | | | |
COMMON NAME (LATIN NAME)	Camphone	Camphor	Fenchone	Menthone	Pinocamphone	Pinocarvone	Thujone	1,8 cineole	Anethole	Carvacrol	Estragol	Eugenol	Fenchole	Methyl chavicol	Thymol	Safrole	Camphene	Limonene	Mycrene	Phellandrene	Pinene	Alpha Terpenene	Azulene	Beta-bisabolene	Beta-caryophellene	Farnasene	Germacrene	Sabinene	Courmarins
Basil, Exotic (*Ocimum basilicum v. basilicum*)		t						t				t		l			t												
Basil, European, sweet (*O. basilicum v. album*)												s		s											s				
Bergamot (*Citrus bergamia*)																	s	s			s								t
Black Pepper (*Piper nigrum*)											s						t	m	s	s	m	t		s	s			s	
Chamomile, German (*Chamomilla recutita*)																							s			s			
Chamomile, Moroccan (*Ormenis mixta*)						t		t				t					s	t	s		m	t		s	s		s	t	
Chamomile, Roman (*Anthemis nobilis*)				m				s									t	t			m	s		s				s	
Clary (*Salvia sclarea*)																		t	t		t								
Cypress (*Cupressus sempervirens*)																	s	s	s		s							s	
Eucalyptus (*Eucalyptus globulus*)						t		l									s	s			m								
Fennel (*Foeniculum vulgare*)		t	t					s	l		s			s		s	s	m			s	t	s						
Frankincense (*Boswellia carteri*)																	m	t	s		m								
Geranium (*Pelargonium graveolens*)																		t	t		t					s		t	
Grapefruit (*Citrus paradisi*)																		l											t
Hyssop (*Hyssopus officinalis*)					m	s		t						t			s	s	s		m						t		
Juniper (*Juniperus communis*)																	s		s		l							m	
Lavandin (*Lavandula hybrida*)		m						s									t	t											t
Lavender (*Lavandula angustifolia*)		t						s									t	t			t					s	s		t
Lemon (*Citrus limon*)																	t	l	t	t	s	t		t	t			t	t
Lemongrass (*Cymbopogon citratus*)																	s	s			t						s		
Marjoram, Spanish (*Thymus mastichina*)	s							l				m		m			t	s	t		s						t	t	
Marjoram, sweet (*Origanum majorana*)		s							t	s	s	s					s	s	s	s							s	m	
Melissa, True (*Melissa officinalis*)																									s				
Neroli (*Citrus aurantium amara*)																		m			m								
Nutmeg (*Myristica fragrans*)								s	(myristicin 5%)			s				t	s	s			t	m	s					m	
Orange, sweet (*C. aurantium sinensis*)																	t	l	t									t	t
Patchouli (*Pogostemon patchouli*)												t					t	t			t	t			s				
Peppermint (*Mentha piperita*)				m				s										s		s	s			t	s				
Petitgrain (*Citrus aurantium amara*)																	s	s											
Pine (*Pinus sylvestris*)								s									s	m	s	s	l				t			t	
Rose Otto (*Rosa centifolia*)								(rose oxide)				t					s	s	s										
Rosemary (*Rosmarinus officinalis*)		s					s	m									s	s			m						s		
Sage (*Salvia officinalis*)		s					m	s								t	s	s	t		s						s		t
Tea Tree (*Melaleuca alternifolia*)								s										t	t	t	s	s					s	t	
Thyme (*Thymus vulgaris – phenols*)										m		or			m		s												
Thyme, sweet (*Thymus vulgaris – alcohols*)																													
Ylang ylang (*Cananga odorata*)										t	s			s							s					s	s		

TABLE 3: List of Oils with Common Name, Latin Name and Plant Family

Common Plant name and Latin name	Family	Page
Angelica *(Angelica archangelica)*	Apiaceae	62
Aniseed *(Pimpinella anisum)*	Apiaceae	66
Basil *(Ocimum basilicum)*	Lamiaceae	75
Benzoin, Siam *(Styrax tonkinensis, Styrax benzoin)*	Styracaceae	94
Bergamot *(Citrus bergamia)*	Rutaceae	92
Black Pepper *(Piper nigrum)*	Piperaceae	87
Cajuput *(Melaleuca leucadendron* or *M. cajuputi)*	Myrtaceae	85
Camphor *(Cinnamomum camphora)*	Lauraceae	81
Caraway *(Carum carvi)*	Apiaceae	63
Carrot seed *(Daucus carota)*	Apiaceae	63
Cedarwood *(Cedrus atlantica)*	Abietaceae	60
Chamomile *(Chamaemelum nobile, Chamomilla recutita* and *Ormenis mixta)*	Asteraceae	67
Cinnamon *(Cinnamomum zeylanicum* or *C. verum)*	Lauraceae	82
Clary *(Salvia sclarea)*	Lamiaceae	79
Clove *(Syzygium aromaticum)*	Myrtaceae	86
Coriander *(Coriandrum sativum)*	Apiaceae	63
Cypress *(Cupressus sempervirens)*	Cupressaceae	70
Dill *(Anethum graveolens)*	Apiaceae	62
Eucalyptus *(Eucalyptus globulus, E. Smithii, E. radiata, E. citriodora)*	Myrtaceae	84
Fennel, sweet *(Foeniculum vulgare* var. *dulce)*	Apiaceae	64
Frankincense *(Boswellia carteri)*	Burseraceae	69
Geranium *(Pelargonium graveolens* and *P. x asperum)*	Geraniaceae	71
Ginger *(Zingiber officinale)*	Zingiberaceae	96
Grapefruit *(Citrus paradisi)*	Rutaceae	92
Hyssop *(Hyssopus officinalis)*	Lamiaceae	72
Jasmine *(Jasminum officinale* var. *grandiflorum)*	Oleaceae	86
Juniper *(Juniperus communis)*	Cupressaceae	71
Lavandin *(Lavandula x intermedia)*	Lamiaceae	74
Lavender *(Lavandula angustifolia, L. vera, L. officinalis)*	Lamiaceae	73
Lemon *(Citrus limon)*	Rutaceae	92
Lemongrass *(Cymbopogon citratus* or *C. flexuosus)*	Poaceae	87
Lemon verbena *(Lippia citriodora)*	Verbenaceae	81
Lime *(Citrus aurantifolia* or *C. limetta)*	Rutaceae	90
Lovage *(Levisticum officinale)*	Apiaceae	65
Mandarin or Tangerine *(Citrus reticulata)*	Rutaceae	93
Marjoram, Spanish *(Thymus mastichina)*	Lamiaceae	80
Marjoram, sweet *(Origanum majorana)*	Lamiaceae	76
Melissa *(Melissa officinalis)*	Lamiaceae	74
Myrrh *(Commiphora myrrha* or *C. molmol)*	Burseraceae	69
Myrtle *(Myrtus communis)*	Myrtaceae	85
Neroli bigarade *(Citrus aurantium* var. *amara* flos*)*	Rutaceae	91
Niaouli *(Melaleuca viridiflora* or *M. quinquenervia)*	Myrtaceae	85
Nutmeg *(Myristica fragrans)*	Myristicaceae	83
Orange, bitter *(Citrus aurantium* var. *amara* per*)*	Rutaceae	90
Orange, sweet *(C. aurantium* var. *sinensis* per*)*	Rutaceae	90
Oregano *(Origanum vulgare)*	Lamiaceae	76
Parsley *(Petroselinum crispum* or *P. sativum)*	Apiaceae	65
Patchouli *(Pogostemon patchouli* or *P. cablin)*	Lamiaceae	76
Peppermint *(Mentha x piperita)*	Lamiaceae	74
Petitgrain bigarde *(Citrus aurantium* var. *amara* fol*)*	Rutaceae	91
Pine *(Pinus sylvestris)*	Abietaceae	61
Rose *(Rosa damascena, R. centifolia)*	Rosaceae	88
Rosemary *(Rosmarinus officinalis)*	Lamiaceae	78
Rosewood *(Aniba rosaeodora)*	Lauraceae	81
Sage *(Salvia officinalis)*	Lamiaceae	78
Sandalwood *(Santalum album)*	Santalaceae	93
Savory *(Satureia montana, Satureia hortensis)*	Lamiaceae	80
Spearmint *(Mentha spicata)*	Lamiaceae	75
Tagetes *(Tagetes glandulifera)*	Asteraceae	68
Tea Tree *(Melaleuca alternifolia)*	Myrtaceae	84
Thyme *(Thymus vulgaris)*	Lamiaceae	80
Valerian *(Valeriana officinalis)*	Valerianaceae	94
Vetiver *(Vetiveria zizanioides)*	Poaceae	88
Ylang ylang *(Cananga odorata)*	Annonaceae	61

4 *Plant Families*

Each plant from which essential oil is derived belongs to one of a number of botanical families. These origins are easy to forget once the oils have been put into little glass bottles. Just as plants show family characteristics in their physical appearance, essential oils show family characteristics in their therapeutic effects, which can be helpful when selecting oils for any particular condition. For would-be therapists, knowledge of the families helps to give a system of, and a pattern for, learning.

Not all plants produce essential oils and of those which do, not all contain a sufficient quantity to justify extraction, either by distillation or solvent extraction. There are well over 200 plants from which essential oils are taken and although most may present possibilities to the perfume industry (also for the study of smell – osmology), not all are popular, free enough from toxicity or necessary for the practice of aromatherapy.

The yield of essential oil from each plant varies not only from year to year in the same country (because of climatic changes), but also from country to country, depending on the growing conditions, so the yields given can only be approximate and are given after the plant name. Those quoted in this chapter have been taken from Guenther (*The Essential Oils*) and *The H&R Book of Perfume*; a 1 per cent yield means that 100 kilos of plant yields approximately 1 litre of essential oil.

There are 21 families which yield the oils used in aromatherapy. Sixteen families yield the most well-known oils; some, like Santalaceae, having hardly any plants in their repertoire and others, like Lamiaceae, having an enormous number.

Unfortunately, botanical names are changed from time to time (which adds to the difficulty of learning them!) Where this is happening, or has happened, all names will be given. Where the common name is almost the same as the Latin name, the former will not be shown.

All plants to be referred to in chapter 5 are entered there under their common name, and this is also the case in all charts, to make them more easily referred to until Latin names become the norm in the UK (see Table 3, page 58, for easy reference).

General properties and effects characteristic to the plant family will be indicated; any special property or effect of note for any particular oil is given in addition to these family traits. Further properties and effects of each oil can be found in the various charts and lists in chapters 3, 6 and 14.

Cautions are given on the results of toxicity tests on *ingestion* by animals, plus the assumption that oils may be wrongly used; these cautions do not necessarily apply to the methods of use (and dilutions used) employed by trained aromatherapists.

Abietaceae (or Pinaceae)

The name Abietaceae is becoming more familiar, though Pinaceae is frequently used. Whichever name is employed, this family, together with the Cupressaceae, belongs to the conifer class.

This is quite a large family, though not many essential oils from its members are in common use.

Family Properties and Effects   Essential oils obtained from the Abietaceae family are highly antiseptic and effective on respiratory disorders involving catarrh.

Cedrus atlantica – wood (cedarwood) 3–5%

See chapter 5 for details on *C. atlantica* and other plants bearing the common name of cedarwood.

Special Properties and Effects   A healing and regenerative oil, *Cedrus atlantica* is a good lymph tonic and is indicated for cellulite. It is useful in cases of oily skin and scalp and has all the family properties too.

Caution   Although the bulk of the oil is composed of terpenes and alcohols, it should be treated with respect, containing as it does around 20 per cent of the ketone atlantone. There seems to be some conflict as to whether or not it is an abortive oil, two authors of well-researched books saying it is and two authors of safety data manuals not mentioning it with respect to toxicity. I suggest it is left alone at the commencement of pregnancy until the baby begins to move (see chapters 5 and 11).

Pinus sylvestris – needles (pine) 0.1–0.5%
This is the species recommended by Valnet; other species of pine are in chapter 5.

Special Properties and Effects   Of the pines, *Pinus sylvestris* has the most comprehensive list of health attributes and is the strongest air antiseptic. It is vaporized in the burns units of some hospitals and has been found to help prevent infection after severe burns. It is an effective expectorant[16] and its antiseptic action is beneficial for almost all respiratory disorders.

Annonaceae

This family contains only one species – *Cananga odorata*, with two varieties, of which ylang ylang is one.

Cananga odorata forma genuina – flowers (ylang ylang) 1.5–2.5%
Alang-ilang in the Philippines implies something fluttering or trembling in a breeze[17] and in Malayan, means 'flower of flowers'. Although harvested throughout the year, the best time to collect the fully developed deep yellow flowers is around May.

Distillation of complete oil of ylang ylang is a long and complicated process, details of which can be found in chapter 5.

Special Properties and Effects   Best quality ylang ylang is an extremely soothing, balancing and calming oil, no doubt due to its high alcohol content (around 50 per cent linalool – this high linalool content is not present in the poorer grades of oil). It is therefore useful in cases of hypertension and tachycardia (rapid heart beat), extreme anxiety, frustration (including sexual) and overwork.

Apiaceae (or Umbelliferae)

Physically, the flower heads of this family resemble umbrellas (which is why I like the name Umbelliferae!) It can be difficult to distinguish one plant in this family from another if you are not a botanist; most of their multi-flowered heads, in shades of off-white or yellow, are similar.

This particular family is regarded as hazardous, many of the oils it produces containing ketones or phenolic ethers, though the evidence is not conclusive regarding ketones – not all are hazardous.

Family Properties and Effects   The Apiaceae family seed oils are extremely balancing to the digestive system (hence their use in aperitifs). Many are also uterine stimulants and may be abortive in action if misused.

Caution   Some contain phenols or ketones and need to be used with care, especially on pregnant women and babies. There is divided opinion regarding the toxicity of carvone (see chapter 3) and until the position is clarified, it may be best to treat all with care (most Apiaceae are best passed on to the public through aromatherapists).

Anethum graveolens – seed (dill) 1.3–1.5%
Dill flowers are not off-white, but bright yellow, the fields presenting an attractive sight.

Special Properties and Effects   Dill seed oil is in babies' gripe water. It helps the flow of bile, thus aiding digestion, and is useful for catarrhal conditions like bronchitis.

Caution   It is believed to be neurotoxic because of its high ketone content (mostly dextro-carvone – yet this can be very low in some dill oils); however, it is also believed that not all carvone molecules are hazardous[18] (see carvone in chapter 3).

Angelica archangelica – seed/roots (angelica) 0.03–0.04%
Although the whole plant is therapeutic, the roots appear to be the part traditionally most used to promote good health. An essential oil it taken from the seeds and both an absolute and an essential oil are produced from the roots. The root oil (most utilized in aromatherapy) contains coumarins, including bergapten (see chapters 3 and 6).

Special Properties and Effects   Angelica's main attribute is its effectiveness against insomnia and nervous exhaustion. It is also a neuro-digestive tonic.

Caution   Because of the coumarin content in both root and seed oils, do not use before ultraviolet exposure.

Carum carvi – seed (caraway) 3–5%
Production of caraway seed oil is increasing, especially in Holland. Here, apart from being exported, the oil is sprayed onto stored potatoes, to prevent them from sprouting. Caraway oil contains the ketone dextro-carvone (up to 50 per cent).

Special Properties and Effects   Its anticatarrhal properties indicate caraway as an excellent oil for the respiratory system and it is one of the best oils for combating vertigo.

Caution   Very few authors consider caraway to be hazardous, even though it contains carvone (see chapter 3). Caraway contains only a trace of the phenolic ether, anethole.

Coriandrum sativum – leaves/seed (coriander) 0.8–1%
Coriander seed oil seems to be one umbellifer which has no known contra-indications against its use, possibly because it has a significant alcohol content (60–80 per cent including linalool – sometimes referred to as coriandrol). The leaf oil (not much used) has an equally significant content of aldehydes.

Special Properties and Effects   Coriander seed oil is anti-inflammatory, relieving rheumatism and arthritis; its antibacterial properties are useful against colds and flu. It is an effective stimulant to the nervous system.

Daucus carota – seed (carrot) 1.5%
The carrot plant grows wild in abundance in France, those with orange roots and those with yellowish-white roots (also used to feed cattle) being cultivated for essential oil. Carrot is possibly the prettiest umbellifer, having earned itself the title of 'Queen Anne's lace'. As the seed begins to form, the head of the plant changes completely, 'fluffing' out and curving inwards – resembling its other common name, 'Bird's Nest'.

Like coriander, carrot oil is high in alcohols (40–60 per cent, mostly carotol). It contains a small amount of asarone (a phenolic ether) but no ketones.

See chapter 8 for fixed oil of carrot.

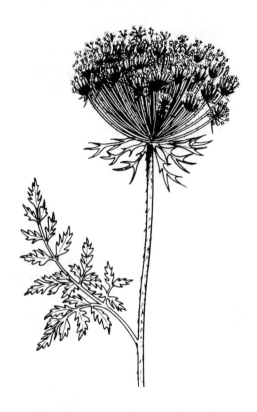

FIGURE 4.1: The early flowering stage of carrot

Special Properties and Effects   Carrot seed oil is tonic and stimulant to both liver and kidneys. Hormonal in action, it helps the pituitary gland to regulate the production of thyroxine and the release of ova. It does not appear to be contra-indicated in pregnancy (perhaps because of its high alcohol content and hormonal action). It is effective on skin complaints such as eczema or a blotchy complexion (as in acne rosacea).

Foeniculum vulgare **var.** *dulce* – seed (sweet fennel) 3–5%
The wild fennel plant and a cultivated sub-species (*capillaceum*) are plants which have been used medicinally for centuries,[19] but these produce bitter

fennel essential oil, not used in aromatherapy. Sweet fennel exists only as a cultivated plant and yields quite a powerful oil, containing a small percentage of the ketone, fenchone, and about 50 per cent of a phenolic ether (trans-anethole). This form of anethole is 15 times less toxic than cis-anethole (see phenols in chapter 3).

Special Properties and Effects   Excellent for the promotion of milk flow in breastfeeding mothers (see chapter 11), it acts as a slight analgesic on muscles. It is helpful for menstrual irregularities and the menopause, due to its hormonal-type action.

Caution   Sweet fennel oil should be treated with respect because of its phenolic content; although not an aggressive oil,[20] it has been suggested as being best not used during pregnancy.

Levisticum officinale – roots (lovage) 0.1–0.6%
An essential oil (reputed to be probably the most powerful natural flavour material ever encountered) is taken from the whole plant (above ground);[21] the roots produce an absolute and an essential oil – the distilled root oil should be chosen for use in aromatherapy.

The plant above ground is credited with being an emmenagogue (mentioned by Mrs Grieve[22] and Richard Mabey[23]). There is no reference to the root oil being emmenagogic in any herbal book of note, or documents on toxicity in the UK or in France. However, it is accredited with this property in one or two modern British and American books on aromatherapy; none says why.

Approximately half the oil is made up of chemicals called phthalides,[24] about which not much is written or known. 3-butylidene phthalide in lovage oil is identical to a lactone found in another oil.[25]

Special Properties and Effects   Detoxifying to the digestive system, lovage root essential oil is stimulating to the excretory and nervous systems, is anticatarrhal and expectorant.

Caution   Lovage root may be a skin sensitizer due to its coumarin content.

Petroselinum crispum or *P. sativum* – leaves/seed (parsley – curly and flat leaved varieties respectively) up to 7% (seed); 0.02–0.3% (leaves)
Parsley, a favourite culinary herb, has an essential oil in both its leaves and its seeds (it can be difficult to ascertain whether leaf oil is exclusively from

the leaves), and an extract can be made from its roots. Parsley is grown extensively in France for the production of dried leaves, which have to be of the highest quality and at their greenest. As a result, essential oil is usually extracted from second grade plants (the quality of the oil is not affected) or from a second cutting when the plants are starting to go to seed (altering the chemical structure of the oil). There is a good market for the seeds for cultivation and the surplus stock of older seeds is used for seed oil, which appears to be the more toxic because of the presence of the phenolic ethers myristicin (a neurotoxic hallucinogen) and apiole (a strong abortifacient). The aroma of the leaf oil (also containing myristicin) is much more like that of the herb itself and it is high in terpenes.

Special Properties and Effects   Parsley leaf, or herb, oil is known mainly for its diuretic properties; it is also antispasmodic.

The seed oil is an emmenagogue, uterine tonic and an effective aid for circulatory troubles connected with menstruation. In strong dosage it is abortive and should not be used by pregnant women.[26]

Caution   Unfortunately, many books give the effects of leaf and seed oil as the same. Also, many suppliers are not certain whether their oil is leaf or seed. Indeed, unless specified, leaf distillation can be from plants with some seed development. Only qualified aromatherapists should use parsley oil and even then, with great respect (there are other oils giving similar effects, which could be used instead).

Pimpinella anisum – seed (aniseed or green aniseed) 2–3%
Two plants have the common name aniseed – the one named above and *Illicium verum* (Chinese star anise – now in many supermarkets), from a totally different family. Three books each give a different name for this family – Illiciaceae, Magnolaceae and Schisandraceae! Both aniseeds appear to yield similar oils chemically, having a high content of the phenolic ether, trans-anethole (sometimes as high as 90 per cent in *Pimpinella anisum*), necessitating care in use, even though *trans*-anethole is less toxic than *cis*-anethole.

Special Properties and Effects   Aniseed oils are antispasmodic, helpful to the respiratory system and stimulant to the reproductive system. Their hormonal action helps to regularize the menstrual cycle and increase the milk flow in breastfeeding women.

Caution   Aniseed should be used with advice from an aromatherapist. It would be prudent not to use either oil on young children or during pregnancy.

Another member of the Illiaceae family, *Illicium lanceolatum*, has as its common name 'Japanese star anise', but this is poisonous.[27]

Asteraceae (or Compositae)

The flowers belonging to this family are daisy-like, each flowerhead being composed of many small flowers rather than petals (hence the name Compositae). Asteraceae may be easier to remember because that favourite and colourful garden flower, the aster, is a member of it. The plants from this family which most interest aromatherapists are the chamomiles, calendula (garden marigold) and tagetes (African marigold).

Family Properties and Effects   The general properties which this family possess are antiseptic, soothing and anti-inflammatory to the skin and digestive system.

Caution   There are 'black sheep' in the Compositae family, as all the artemisias, most of which are neurotoxic, belong to it. Because of their relatively high ketone or phenolic ether content artemisia oils are available in France only from pharmacies: wormwood (*Artemisia absinthium* – thujone); mugwort (*Artemisia vulgaris* – thujone), also known as armoise; tarragon (*Artemisia dracunculus* – estragole) are not generally used in aromatherapy in the UK and should not be made generally available.

Chamaemelum nobile, Chamomilla recutita and *Ormenis mixta* –
flowerheads (chamomile) 1–1.7%
(See chapter 5 for other names for, and botanical differences between, these essential oils.)

Chamomile plants contain a colourless compound which decomposes during distillation to produce azulene, changing to a blue colour in the process.

Special Properties and Effects   Because of its higher azulene content *Chamomilla recutita* is the most efficient in treating irritable or inflamed skin conditions. *Chamaemelum nobile* (containing a significant amount of esters) is favoured for gout sufferers and is undoubtedly the choice for children. *Ormenis mixta*, perhaps preferable for depression,[28]

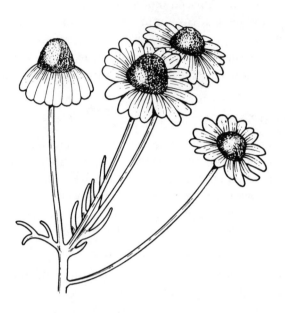

FIGURE 4.2: German chamomile *(Chamomilla recutita)*

contains more alcohols, and is sometimes called the poor man's Roman chamomile as its price is lower.

Tagetes glandulifera – flowers (tagetes) 0.2–0.4%

Tagetes is sometimes confused with calendula as both possess the common name of 'marigold' (chapter 5). It contains approximately 35–50 per cent of tagetone, a ketone, and its coumarin content makes it a photo-sensitizer (see chapter 6).

Special Properties and Effects   Effective on slow-to-heal wounds, burns and bruises, it is also useful against catarrhal conditions. Competent on fungal infections of the feet and of the digestive system (candida), it may also promote the onset of menstruation.[29] It is an excellent deterrent to houseflies!

Caution   Being neurotoxic, it should be used in a controlled manner; it is not recommended for use on pregnant women or on children without advice. Do not use immediately before exposure to the sun or sunbeds.

Burseraceae

The two oils of interest to aromatherapists in this family (frankincense and myrrh) are available distilled or as resins – for aromatherapy the distilled oils should be used.

Family Properties and Effects   They are expectorant and helpful to bronchitis. Both are invaluable for healing wounds and ulcers, promoting, and afterwards reducing, scar tissue.

Boswellia carteri – resin (frankincense or olibanum) 5%
Boswellia carteri is the species most used for the extraction of the resin from which the essential oil is distilled. The resin is a pathogenic exudation for defence when strips are peeled from the inner bark, and some people may not be comfortable with the idea of using such a product for healing purposes. A milky fluid runs down the tree after the first cut, but is not used. After repeated strips are removed, large clear globules (collected for distillation or solvent extraction) begin to form. Yellowy or clear 'tears' generally (though not always) produce a higher quality oil than that from the orangey red ones.

Special Properties and Effects   Both relaxing and antidepressive, distilled frankincense is an emotionally balancing oil with the added quality of being an immunostimulant.[30]

Commiphora myrrha or *C. molmol* – resin (myrrh) 6–8%
The resin in myrrh, unlike that of frankincense, occurs naturally, but the yield, dark yellow to reddish brown lumps rather than tears, is increased by making incisions in the bark. These are distilled to obtain a yellowy orange essential oil or treated by solvent extraction to produce a dark orangey brown resinoid – poor quality ones being somewhat sticky.

Special Properties and Effects   The distilled oil is antifungal and useful against candida, in the mouth and vagina, and athlete's foot. Myrrh is cooling and moisturizing to the skin, and anti-inflammatory. Being hormone-like, it is said to be helpful in balancing the production of thyroxine and is reputed to diminish the sexual appetite.[31]

Nowhere in any of my many reference books can I find reference to myrrh being an emmenagogue, nor in Richard Mabey's well-researched book on herbs;[32] one or two British writers have recommended that it should not be used in pregnancy (without saying why). As it has hormonal properties, it could, like rose otto, be a balancing oil to the reproductive system, rather than an emmenagogue. During all the publicity about essential oils and toxicity, begun in 1991, not one newspaper has been interested in publishing positive facts, so I welcome the opportunity to suggest that perhaps after all, myrrh may be innocent.

Compositae, see Asteraceae.

Cupressaceae

This family, like that of Abietaceae, belongs to the Conifer class. The two oils concerning us from this family are cypress and juniper.

Family Properties and Effects   Both contain roughly 70 per cent monoterpenes, around 40 per cent of which is pinene. Both oils reduce nervous tension, help stress-related conditions and insomnia, are anti-rheumatic, astringent – balancing to an oily skin – and help reduce cellulite.

Cupressus sempervirens – flowers/leaves (cypress) 1.3–1.5%
Cypress is distilled mainly from the leaves and twigs, though occasionally the flowers or cones are included, depending when the trees are pruned. Originating in eastern Mediterranean countries, distillation was once concentrated in the south of France.[33]

Special Properties and Effects   Its astringent qualities are its main asset, making cypress useful against bed-wetting[34] and 'hot flushes', especially if used regularly as a preventive measure. The reduction of menopausal tension is the main effect of its calming properties. Its anti-spasmodic action makes it effective when inhaled during an asthma attack.

Caution   Anyone with excessive high blood pressure should not use this oil on a regular basis – due to its astringent properties (the cones increase these).

Juniperus communis – berries (juniper) 0.2–1.6%
The yield from juniper berries alone is 28–30%, but the price is still relatively high as the berries take a long time to pick. Details of the two distinct qualities of oil from this small tree can be found in chapter 5.

Special Properties and Effects   Juniperberry oil is stimulating to the circulatory, excretory, digestive and respiratory systems – a tonic to the heart, diuretic and anti-inflammatory to the digestive tract (including the pancreas, therefore useful in diabetes).

Caution   Do not confuse with *Juniperus sabina*, both the plant and essential oil of which are abortive (see chapter 5). *J. communis* is not an emmenagogue. It has been suggested that, because of its strong diuretic effects, it may be best not to use it in the first few months of pregnancy, and although it appears as such in *Aromatherapy for Common Ailments*, I was asked to be especially cautious in that book, as it was written primarily for the American market.

Geraniaceae

Of the Pelargonium genus in this very small family, the species *graveolens* is the one used to extract oil for aromatherapy. The fact that the common name, rose geranium, is sometimes used causes some confusion (see chapter 5).

Pelargonium graveolens and *P. x asperum* – leaves (geranium) 0.1–0.2%
(Réunion and French); 1.2–1.5% (Moroccan and Egyptian)

Special Properties and Effects   High in alcohols and containing a sizeable proportion of esters, geranium is a therapeutically kind oil. Anti-inflammatory, it is soothing and cooling to the skin – helping a multitude of skin conditions including chilblains. It is stimulant to the liver and pancreas, therefore helpful to diabetes and is a generally balancing oil to the nervous system, especially for agitation.

Graminae, see Poaceae.

Lamiaceae or Labiatae

The largest of all the plant families concerning us, it contains all the well-known herbs – including lavender.

All labiates are renowned for their penetrating aroma, no doubt due to the fact that the essential oil is stored on the surface of the leaves and is easily released.

Family Properties and Effects   The majority of labiate oils are without any hazards or major contra-indications. Many are helpful for headaches, nasal congestion and various muscular problems, each oil giving its own specific aid – analgesic, anti-inflammatory, etc. As a general rule, these very aromatic labiates are stimulating (lavender is more sedative), bringing vigour and energy to the body as a whole, or to one particular system, e.g. the respiratory system. The family is not a simple one as some members contain more alcohols, some more aldehydes and one or two need care in use.

Hyssopus officinalis – flowers/leaves (hyssop) 0.7–1%
It was interesting to discover that hyssop flowers all grow on the same side of the stem – a fact I did not notice until we actually grew a field of it.

This beautiful aromatic plant is one labiate whose oil needs to be used carefully; it is neurotoxic, containing a significant percentage of pinocamphone (a ketone). In France, it can only be purchased from a pharmacy. For the trained therapist, it is a most useful oil and properly used, can be very beneficial.

Special Properties and Effects   Anti-inflammatory, hyssop is helpful to asthma, cystitis and a sore throat. It is excellent in alleviating the aggravation caused by scratching eczema. It is indicated for ovarian problems at puberty.[35]

Caution   Although its pinocamphone content makes it contra-indicated for those predisposed to epilepsy, I have used it in minute concentration on an epileptic friend, with positive results, though I do not necessarily recommend that you follow this example. As always, it is a question of the dose, and the theory of a 'homoeopathic' percentage is a good principle where powerful oils are concerned.

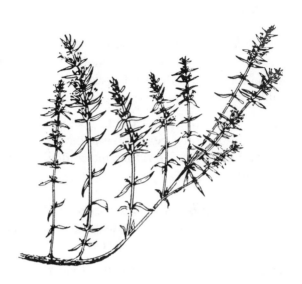

FIGURE 4.3: Hyssop

It is interesting that *Hyssopus officinalis* var. *decumbens* is low in ketones and high in oxides, and is noted as having no known contra-indications.[36]

Lavandula angustifolia, L. vera, L. officinalis – flowers/leaves (lavender)
1–1.5%
Although I would like the name *L. vera* to be kept for wild lavender, these species are one and the same; all yield what is known as true or 'fine' lavender (growing in the wild or as cultivated plants).[37] As a commercial proposition wild lavender is not viable as the quantities required to meet demand are not available and the price in any case, would be horrendous! (See chapter 5.)

Special Properties and Effects   The main attributes of lavender are its gentleness and effectiveness, making it an oil suitable for all ages, from babies to senior citizens. Used mostly for its ability to ease stress and relieve headaches and insomnia, it is the most used oil, including use in hospitals where it is used almost exclusively compared with other essential oils. It is interesting to note that lavender is classed as a non-toxic oil and is even used neat in an emergency such as a burn, yet Culpeper's

Herbal says of lavender: 'Caution is needed when using the essential oil, as it is extremely potent'!

Lavandula x *intermedia* – flowers/leaves (lavandin) 1.8–2.5%

Lavandin, of which there are many varieties, is often used to adulterate true lavender (or even sold *as* lavender). The aroma, though more camphoraceous, is quite lavender-like and pleasant. (See chapter 5.)

Special Properties and Effects   Because of its camphor content, it is a good oil for muscular, respiratory and circulatory problems which can be helped by camphor, and is the preferred oil of the two (see camphor, and chapter 5).

Melissa officinalis – leaves (melissa) 0.01%

True melissa oil has limited availability and confusion arises because of a mixed oil, also named melissa (see chapter 5).

Special Properties and Effects   True melissa is exceptionally calming for hysteria and is one of the best oils for pregnancy sickness. It is good for vertigo and, according to a reliable French work published in 1990, is not contra-indicated for pregnant women. It is a good antiviral oil against herpes simplex I (cold sore).

Mentha x *piperita* – leaves (peppermint) 0.3–1%

In America peppermint oil has many applications in the food and tobacco industries and there are strict rules about how the oil should be rectified or folded (see chapter 2). Outside the USA (the largest producer of *Mentha* x *piperita*), peppermint (often from *Mentha arvensis*) is also frequently rectified – see chapter 5 – so that the active part, menthol (initially around 80 per cent), is decreased in proportion (see chapter 5). As the food and tobacco industries buy peppermint oil by the tens of tons, it is difficult to find a non-rectified or non-folded oil and hazards attributed to peppermint are likely to stem from these oils. We feel it important to buy our *Mentha* x *piperita* direct from the distiller to be certain of obtaining an oil that has not been folded or altered in any way.

Special Properties and Effects   Essentially a cooling and anti-inflammatory oil, peppermint is credited with being helpful for irritable bowel syndrome[38] and with stimulating the ovaries.[39] Perhaps it is due to this latter effect that it is thought to be contra-indicated during pregnancy, though Franchomme does not give it as such. It usually contains no (or only a trace of) pulegone, the ketone responsible for labelling pennyroyal (which contains over 50 per cent) as an abortive oil. Peppermint oil contains a varying percentage of the ketone menthone.

Caution   As peppermint oil is powerful, it should be used in very low concentrations and not on very young children, as it may cause irritation. Otherwise, there are no known contra-indications to the complete oil. Should a folded oil be purchased, any powerful components would obviously be considerably increased as a percentage of the total oil.

Mentha spicata – leaves (spearmint) 0.5–0.8%

This plant originated in Europe and when introduced into America, the essential oil became one of their most important flavourings (for chewing gum, of course!) You may have experienced in North Africa the strong spearmint tea, made from *Mentha viridis*, which is always offered to visitors. Spearmint oil is mostly produced for the flavour industry and not used so much in aromatherapy – a pity, because I love the aroma.

Special Properties and Effects   It is reported to be antispasmodic, carminative and stimulant, as well as being, like peppermint, a good digestive stimulant. It is useful as an inhalation against respiratory disorders (including the common cold at its first stages) as it is anti-inflammatory, decongestant and anticatarrhal. The not-so-powerful aroma makes it particularly suitable for children suffering from colds, nausea, or other digestive problems.

Caution   Spearmint oil is contra-indicated in pregnancy,[40] no doubt because of the ketone content (it contains up to 60 or 70 per cent of laevo-carvone). It is not a skin irritant, nor is it a sensitizer nor phototoxic;[41] nevertheless, it may be neurotoxic and abortive and should be used with care until the carvone question has been thoroughly researched (see chapter 3).

Ocimum basilicum – leaves (basil) 0.1–0.2%

Because of confusion over possible hazards, details on this much maligned but extremely useful essential oil can be found in chapter 5.

Special Properties and Effects Basil is a good all-round oil for most circulation and heart problems, including arteriosclerosis, hypotension, tachycardia, irregular heart beat and varicose veins; it is also useful against cramp. Stimulating and warming, it is indicated for uterine congestion and may also be helpful for period pains.

Origanum majorana – leaves (marjoram or sweet marjoram) 0.5–2%
Thymus mastichina, on account of its common name (Spanish marjoram), is mostly incorrectly credited with the therapeutic effects of *Origanum majorana*, and both oils are sold as marjoram (see chapter 5).

Special Properties and Effects Like basil, sweet marjoram is indicated for tachycardia and is a cardiovascular oil. It is very useful for controlling nervous excitement, agitation and obsessions (possibly indicating its use for the oversexed![42]) (For the effects of Spanish marjoram see *Thymus mastichina* later in this section.)

Origanum vulgare L. – leaves (oregano) 0.07–0.4%
Origanum vulgare L. contains up to 7 per cent thymol (a phenol), whereas *O. vulgare* L. var. *viride (virens)* can contain up to 50 per cent of this same chemical. We try to purchase only the low-thymol variety, as the other is a skin irritant.

Special Properties and Effects Said to stimulate the appetite, oregano also stimulates the menstrual flow. It helps to relieve the pain in rheumatism and, being an expectorant, it is helpful for asthma, bronchitis and coughs.

Caution Unless it is known what type of oregano you are buying, it is best to seek the advice of an aromatherapist before using.

Pogostemon patchouli and *P. cablin* – leaves (patchouli) 2–3%
Very important to perfumery, patchouli is not among the top ten oils used in aromatherapy. The synthetic aroma used to be a favourite; when we first had our aromatherapy shop in the 1970s we were continually asked only for patchouli, but we were not selling any because the genuine oil was not recognized, and regarded as too expensive!

The leaves, cut every few months, attain their highest oil content in the three pairs of newest leaves. Cutting is therefore aimed at a growth of five pairs, as the essential oil content of larger leaves is negligible. Patchouli is an excellent natural fixative – a good friend to anyone wishing to create a long-lasting perfume without the use of synthetics.

Approximately half the oil consists of sesquiterpenes, not possessing great therapeutic value; around 40 per cent is made up of various alcohols, patchoulol being the main one.

Special Properties and Effects   It is very effective in healing cracked and broken skin,[43] due to its regenerative properties. It is anti-inflammatory, bactericidal and is a useful oil generally for improving the skin, including cellulite conditions. It is an emotionally balancing oil, non-irritant and non-toxic.[44]

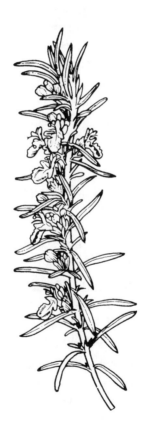

FIGURE 4.4: Rosemary

Rosmarinus officinalis – flowering tops (rosemary) 1–2%
Rosemary (the oil is distilled from the flowering tops) is one of a number of plants which have several chemotypes; in this case, *camphor, cineole* and *verbenone*. All chemotypes are named after the main chemical constituent. Rosemary oils available to aromatherapists at the moment all contain varying amounts of 1,8-cineole and camphor, which variation renders rosemary open to easy adulteration. 1,8-cineole is easily removed from *Eucalyptus globulus*, and camphor from *Cinnamomum camphora*, at very low cost – both are often used as adulterants in rosemary oils.

Special Properties and Effects   Chemotypes with a high camphor content are more effective in cases of rheumatism and fluid retention but otherwise many of the effects overlap, including the uplifting of the spirits and the stimulation of the mind. Rosemary is helpful against fainting and bedwetting[45] (this reference does not state a particular chemotype).

Caution   The verbenone chemotype is the one which is best not used in pregnancy, and should not be used on children[46] because this particular ketone is neurotoxic. The cineole chemotype does not present these hazards.[47]

Salvia officinalis – dried leafy stems (sage) 1–2%
Sage is distilled from the leaves preferably before the plant flowers, or after the flowers have died. The latter oil contains more ketones. It should not be confused with *Salvia sclarea*, which is a different species (see chapter 5). Sage contains significant amounts of ketones (mainly thujone), whereas clary's strength is in its ester and alcohol content.

Special Properties and Effects   Sage oil has been found to be helpful in all cases of congestion, such as bronchitis, fluid retention, period pains etc. It is also effective against both viral infection of the stomach and the virus responsible for glandular fever.

Caution   Because of its high thujone content (up to and around 60 per cent), until more is known about the different thujones (see chapter 3) sage oil may need care in use, being best used under the direction of an aromatherapist (the oil is sold only through pharmacies in France).

Salvia sclarea – dried stems with flowers and leaves (clary) under 1%

This beautiful, strongly aromatic plant (the aroma from one stem alone can fill a whole house) can grow to a height of up to 5 feet (1.5 metres) and has several flowering bracts on one stem. It is cut after the flowers have died and is often dried before distilling. I prefer clary sage to be called 'clary' (I have referred to it as such in this book), to save confusion with sage oil, as it is often (incorrectly) used in place of it.

Special Properties and Effects   Because of its oestrogen-like properties (possibly due to the presence of sclareol – an alcohol), clary oil is good for women's hormonal problems.[48] Although particularly helpful in lack of, or irregular menstruation, it is possibly on account of the hormonal effect that the oil is sometimes given as contra-indicated during early pregnancy. Clary is extremely valuable for balancing emotions.[49]

Caution   Drinking alcohol before or after using clary can increase the effects of the alcohol.

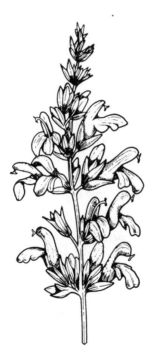

FIGURE 4.5: Clary

Satureia montana and *Satureia hortensis* – leaves (mountain and summer savory respectively) approx. 0.2%

Savory is recommended for use only by trained aromatherapists because of its high carvacrol content (around 40 per cent), a phenol which is a skin irritant if not correctly diluted.

Special Properties and Effects   Tests have been carried out at the Scottish Agricultural College which show the power of *Satureia hortensis* as an effective bactericide,[50] and it is known also as a powerful antifungal and antiviral agent. It is reputed to be a sexual tonic.

Thymus mastichina – flowering tops (Spanish/wild marjoram) 1.2% minimum

Because the use of this oil is confused with that of *Origanum majorana*, it is discussed in more detail in chapter 5.

Special Properties and Effects   Bactericidal and expectorant, Spanish marjoram is indicated in sinus and catarrhal cases, including bronchitis.[51] Some people have tried, without success, to use this oil to reduce sexual activity; in fact it is *Origanum majorana* which is credited with this effect, indicating yet again the importance of using Latin names.

Caution   Because of the high 1,8-cineole content, use with care.

Thymus vulgaris – flowering tops 0.7–1% (red – ct. phenol); 0.3–0.8% (sweet – ct. alcohol)

The chemotypes of essential oil from *Thymus vulgaris* plants grown from seed, or collected in the wild, are very diverse in their properties. They fall into two main groups, 'phenolic' thymes being skin irritant and 'sweet' thymes (those containing alcohols) being without hazard – even on children (see chapter 5).

Special Properties and Effects of Phenolic Thymes   Red thymes are strongly anti-infectious, therefore extremely useful in cases of colds, flu, sore throat, etc. Good general tonics, they are effective in severe cases of depression.[52]

Caution They are irritant to the skin because of their high phenol content – and because they need to be used with care their use is best left to aromatherapists.

Special Properties and Effects of Sweet Thymes   Sweet thymes have alcohol as their main constituent, and are antibacterial and anti-fungal (which makes them useful against *Candida albicans* – thrush). They have good tonic effects on the nervous system and are immunostim-ulant. They are indicated for bronchitis, cystitis, rheumatism and vaginitis and can be helpful in cases of dry eczema. Thyme was used after World War II in Germany on children with low immune systems; it gave them a will to live and an appetite.[53]

Lauraceae

For a family containing oils such as sassafras, cassia and camphor (from the wood), which present hazards, it is surprising to see in it the gentle *Aniba rosaeodora*.

Family Properties and Effects   Practically the whole of this family are antifungal, bactericidal, antiviral and either tonic or stimulant.

Aniba rosaeodora – wood (rosewood or bois-de-rose) 0.8–1.6%
Rosewood oil is a tender subject for ecologists and as it may come from more than one source, more details can be found in chapter 5.

Special Properties and Effects   One of the main uses of *Aniba rosaeodora* is for its effect upon the nervous system, where it acts as a tonic in depressed states. Because of its high linalool content, it is helpful in skin care and general and sexual fatigue.[54]

Cinnamomum camphora – leaves/wood (camphor) average 1.5%
I am not very happy about the use of *C. camphora* wood oil in aromatherapy as it is a fractionated oil (see chapter 2). It is also highly unlikely that anyone buying this oil even receives essential oil (see chapter 5), as most white camphor today is synthesized from the terpene alpha-pinene. The effects of this oil should not be confused with those of *Dryobalanops camphora* (Borneo camphor) from the Dipterocarpaceae family (see chapter 5).

The essential oil from the *leaves* is reminiscent of rosewood oil (see chapter 5).

Special Properties and Effects   Camphor is a tonic and general stimulant. It is analgesic, therefore helpful to rheumatic pain and is indicated for chronic bronchitis.

Caution   Camphor as available at the moment can be over-stimulant to the heart in high doses; it is also neurotoxic and abortive.

Cinnamomum zeylanicum or *Cinnamomum verum* – bark/leaves
(cinnamon) 0.5–1% (bark); 1.6–1.8% (leaves)
Although there are several types of cinnamon trees, only two yield true cinnamon oil; those from Sri Lanka producing the oil with the best aroma.

Bark and leaf each contain an essential oil, one slightly different from the other.

Leaf oil contains a high percentage of the phenol eugenol (around 80 per cent), whereas bark oil is almost equally high in an aldehyde called cinnamaldehyde. Both chemicals are hazardous in their own way if the oils are used in excess or incorrectly.

Bark: Cinnamic aldehyde, when isolated from the whole oil, is a severe skin irritant; the whole bark oil does not appear to be so (see chapter 6).

Leaf: This has a higher content of kinder constituents like alcohols and esters than bark oil, which suggests it may be a slightly less hazardous oil to use, though I feel that the phenol content (eugenol) could present an irritant hazard equal to that of the cinnamic aldehyde in the bark oil.

Joint Properties and Effects   Both oils are efficient bactericidal agents, are antifungal and antiviral.

Special Properties and Effects of Cinnamon Bark Oil   Bark oil is a good general tonic, especially to the reproductive system – where it is a sexual tonic; effective for stimulating menstruation and helping uterine contractions during birth.[55]

Caution   In too concentrated a mix and used too regularly, cinnamon bark oil is a sensitizer; it can also be over-stimulating to the nervous system; it is best not used in early pregnancy or on young children.

Special Properties and Effects of Cinnamon Leaf Oil   The leaf oil is not attributed with any effects on the menstrual system and it is an immunostimulant. It is indicated for sleepiness – perhaps a good oil to include in an inhalation mix for car drivers on a long journey.

Caution   The leaf oil is also irritant on sensitive skins and mucous surfaces because of the phenol content and should be used with care. Both bark and leaf oil are best used under the direction of an aromatherapist.

Myristicaceae

Myristica fragrans – fruit (nutmeg) 5–15%

Two essential oils are produced from the fruit of this tree – nutmeg and mace. Mace is the thin, lacy covering around the nutmeg 'seed', removed before the nutmeg is sold for cooking purposes. There is little oil of mace produced, as the perfume industry no longer distinguishes between the two oils. The therapeutic effects of the two are the same.

Special Properties and Effects   The phenolic ether content of nutmeg oil (mainly myristicin) must be noted because, although only present in a small amount (4–6 per cent) it is a very powerful brain stimulant (a hallucinogen) and a tonic to the uterus. When dilute and used now and again with care nutmeg oil can aid muscular aches and pains and insomnia, due to its analgesic effect. My grandmother used to grate nutmeg on the top of bedtime cocoa to ensure a good night's sleep.

Caution   Used incorrectly and in excessive amounts, nutmeg can cause the mind to 'float', producing hallucinations. To be used with care and not until the end of pregnancy, nutmeg oil is best left for use by a competent aromatherapist.

Myrtaceae

The essential oils of this family are mostly from eucalyptus and melaleuca trees. In both cases the oil is found in little pockets inside the leaves, which need to be broken to release the aroma.

Family Properties and Effects   All are highly antiseptic, tonic and stimulant, being useful for infections of varying degrees, particularly of the respiratory system.

Caution   Most Myrtaceae contain a significant amount of 1,8-cineole (an oxide which can sting open wounds) so should be treated with respect.

Eucalyptus globulus, E. smithii, E. radiata, E. citriodora – leaves
(eucalyptus) 3–4.5%; 3–4.5% (cineole type); 0.5–2% respectively

There are several species of eucalyptus (over 200!) and the differences between these four appear in chapter 5.

Special Properties and Effects   All four are indicated for urinary tract infections. Particular effects of note – *E. globulus* is antifungal, *E. smithii* is antiviral and expectorant, *E. citriodora* is indicated for hyper-tension, and both it and *E. radiata* are anti-inflammatory, making them useful for rheumatoid arthritis. *E. radiata* is especially helpful in reducing inflammation and in cases of endometriosis.

Caution   *E. globulus* is rather strong for very young children or babies as it is often rectified – *E. smithii* is an excellent substitute.[56] *E. citriodora* should be used well diluted on people with sensitive skin because of the aldehyde content (citronellal).

Melaleuca alternifolia – leaves (tea tree) 10–15%
All melaleuca trees come under the general heading of 'tea tree', *Melaleuca alternifolia* and *Melaleuca linariifolia* being known only by that name. The latter species yields an oil with strong camphor and eucalyptus tendencies in the aroma and is less warmly aromatic than *M. alternifolia*. Tea tree oil has been given a great deal of publicity and can be used directly on the skin and mucous surfaces quite safely.

My husband still has niggling doubts as to the authenticity of all tea tree oils; undoubtedly there is a synthetic tea tree oil on the market, but how genuine is the genuine article? As he is told that the trees have grown from seed and are not cloned, and as the 1,8-cineole content from a genuine oil can be as high as 80 per cent, he wonders: do the trees from seeds obligingly produce an oil low enough in cineole to give the claimed maximum in a genuine oil of 15 per cent?

Special Properties and Effects   Tea tree oil is antiviral, antifungal and anti-inflammatory; many of its attributes, including its immunostimulant effects, are no doubt due to its extremely powerful bactericidal properties. Applied before radiotherapy, it has been used to protect the skin from the deep burning effects.[57]

Melaleuca leucadendron or *M. cajuputi* – leaves (cajuput or white tea tree) 0.8–1%

In the Philippines 'kaju-puti' means 'white wood'.[58] Each country or area seems to have its own panacea for most problems; if enough research were done it may be discovered that tea tree and lavender are not the only 'use it for everything' essential oils. We have found cajuput, geranium and lemon oils to be equally all-embracing. The 1,8-cineole content in cajuput is 14–65 per cent, but the oil seems to be without hazard when employed in a controlled manner (see Synergy in chapter 6).

Special Properties and Effects   Used in the Far East for colds, sore throats and headaches, cajuput has proved its ability in these respects in other countries. It is useful in cases of rheumatoid arthritis, varicose veins, sinusitis and gastric problems.

Melaleuca viridiflora or *M. quinquenervia* – leaves (niaouli) 0.6–1.5%

As this tree grows wild in abundance, it does not need to be cultivated. The oil resembles that of cajuput, containing up to 65 per cent of 1,8-cineole. The genuine oil is difficult to come by so buy from a specialist aromatherapy supplier.

Special Properties and Effects   Due to its decongestant properties, niaouli has been found helpful not only to catarrhal conditions, but also to haemorrhoids, thread veins and varicose veins and several digestive problems. It is a hormonal balancer and provides protection against deep burning in radiography. Niaouli is anti-inflammatory and as such is helpful against rheumatism and arthritis.[59]

Myrtus communis – flowers/leaves/twigs (myrtle) 0.1–0.5%

Myrtle grows wild in the countries round the Mediterranean, the essential oil being extracted mainly from the twigs and aromatic leaves – occasionally the sweet-smelling flowers are included.

Special Properties and Effects   The oil from myrtle resembles that of niaouli, including the 1,8-cineole content. Its effects on the body are almost identical (perhaps not quite so comprehensive); it is also hormonal.

Syzygium aromaticum or *Eugenia caryophyllata* – bud/leaf (clove) 15% (bud); 2–3% (leaf)

Like several plants in the essential oil world, the clove tree produces more than one essential oil; the differences can be found in chapter 5.

Special Properties and Effects   Well known for its analgesic virtues (used in dentistry), clove bud has also proved useful for shingles, multiple sclerosis and prickly heat. It is an excellent uterine tonic helping to relax both these muscles and the mind.[60] According to research done, there are no known contra-indications to date when used carefully.

Caution   Clove bud oil should be used with respect, i.e. in moderation with regard to length of time used and dose. In concentrated form, it may irritate both skin and mucous surfaces due to its phenol content (eugenol), but careful use, well diluted or used in conjunction with other oils, should not present any hazards.

Oleaceae

Jasminum officinale var. *grandiflorum* or *J. officinale* – flowers (jasmine)

Although not an essential oil, this absolute is a well-loved aroma and it is important to understand the huge variance in quality of this and other exotic absolutes:

'Jasmine absolute is frequently adulterated. Its high cost seems to tempt certain suppliers and producers beyond their moral resistance.'

Steffen Arctander, who was a respected authority on essential oils and perfume materials, lists all the possible adulterants, including ylang ylang fractions. Benzyl acetate (which occurs naturally in jasmine), the synthetic substitute of which costs one hundredth of the price of jasmine, is also used to 'regulate' the price of jasmine absolute, which can vary by more than £1000 per kilo between the many qualities available on the market! (See chapter 2.) A synthetic called jasmone (with a similar aroma to jasmine) is often sold as jasmine.

Pinaceae, see Abietaceae

Piperaceae

Piper nigrum – berries (black pepper) 2%

Black pepper is an attractive climbing plant and the berries are picked before they have completely ripened. They are then left to dry in the sun, when they turn black, being ground before distillation commences. Black pepper is composed mostly of monoterpenes (about 70 per cent) and sesquiterpenes (about 25 per cent, of which beta-caryophyllene is the major one).

Special Properties and Effects   The oil is anticatarrhal and stimulant to the circulatory and digestive systems as well as to the sexual appetite. Being analgesic it is indicated for toothache. Its anticatarrhal and expectorant properties make it useful for respiratory disorders.

Poaceae (or Graminae)

Although the two plants concerning us are grasses, one oil is distilled from the grass and the other from the roots.

Family Properties and Effects   The generic traits of oils from this family are their effects on acne, aches and pains and the circulation (where they act as stimulants).

Cymbopogon citratus or *C. flexuosus* – grass (lemongrass) 1.8–2.2%

The first species is sometimes given the common name of citronella – although citronella is in fact *Cymbopogon nardus*, another species of the same family. This last contains many more alcohols (up to 65 per cent geraniol) and far fewer aldehydes (up to 15 per cent citronellal). Lemongrass contains up to 70–85 per cent aldehydes (citrals – mostly neral and geranial).

Distilled from the grass, lemongrass oil has one of the strongest aromas: even one drop in a blend is unmistakable. It has quite a strong colour and can leave a bright yellow mark on some fabrics. In the perfume world it is used mainly for the isolation of citral.

Special Properties and Effects   Lemongrass is a good head clearer and 'wake up' oil for first thing in the morning. Its tonic effects are useful on cellulite and on the digestive system. It is an excellent insect repellent.[61]

Caution   It should never be used neat on the skin because of its possible irritant properties (due mainly to the citral content); however, when diluted in a carrier, it is without hazard except on sensitive skins. Treat with respect.

Vetiveria zizanioides – roots (vetiver) 2–3%
Vetiver has been introduced into some volcanic and also mountainous countries to help control soil erosion.

Essential oil of vetiver is distilled from the dried and chopped rootlets of this grass, and its ester content makes it an effective oil therapeutically and also one of the best fixatives for use in perfumery.

Special Properties and Effects   Renowned for its relaxing effects on the nervous system, it stimulates pancreatic secretions, which may indicate its use on people suffering from diabetes. It is also indicated for sluggish periods.

Rosaceae

Small but very prestigious, this family has the queen of flowers, the rose, as one of its members. More must have been written on rose than any other oil and it is surely the best known, and possibly the oldest, perfume.

There are two main rose species used nowadays both for distillation (when the oil is referred to as rose otto) and for solvent extraction (when the result is an absolute). The species *alba* and *gallica* are no longer used.

Rosa centifolia – petals (Moroccan or Indian rose or cabbage rose) 0.02–0.05%
This light pink cabbage rose, with three times as many petals as the Bulgarian species, is cultivated for both distillation and solvent extraction. The absolute is called 'rose de mai' and the plant was first cultivated in France, though now, Morocco produces much of the world requirement. The yield of oil from the cabbage type rose is higher than that from the Bulgarian rose.

The essential oil from the cabbage rose is usually referred to simply as rose oil, or if from Morocco, Moroccan rose otto. The name 'otto' is generally reserved for the distilled oil from the damascena rose. I prefer to call both distilled oils 'otto', to save confusion with the absolute oils.

Rosa damascena – petals (Bulgarian or Turkish rose) 0.01–0.03%
Originally *Rosa damascena* was probably a hybrid of *Rosa gallica* L. and *Rosa canina* L.[62] though it can now be found growing wild in various countries.

This beautiful deep pink multi-petalled rose gives the original and most valued rose otto (or attar, from the Persian *'atir*, meaning perfumed) and the most coveted oil comes from Bulgaria. The same rose is also used for the production of an absolute.

The distilled oils contain a significant amount of the alcohol citronellol (from 40 per cent to as high as 60 per cent in Bulgarian oil), with low phenyl ethyl alcohol (PEA) content. Absolutes contain about 50 per cent PEA oil (thus both are open to adulteration with synthetic PEA) and much less citronellol; the effects are therefore different. N.B. When isolated, PEA is toxic by inhalation and is often the cause of asthmatic – and skin – reactions to artificially scented household products, such as pot pourri and cleaning sprays.[63]

Absolutes have a sweeter, richer and headier aroma than distilled oils, as larger molecules (including colour molecules) than those which are volatile can escape into the solvent used. The properties and effects given below are for distilled oils only.

Special Properties and Effects Rose otto has many attributes – if only it were less expensive! It is a wonderful oil for women at all times and is gentle enough to be used on children.

It balances the hormones and therefore regulates the periods; it is therefore mistakenly quoted as an oil to avoid in the first few months of pregnancy. Dr Dietrich Wabner, a professor at Munich University researching essential oils and an expert on rose oil, tells me it is not an emmenagogue but enables menstruation to occur in a regular and normal fashion by influencing the hormones.[64]

Rose otto is an excellent oil for the skin, helping to prevent wrinkles, reduce broken veins and ease dermatitis and eczema. It is indicated for chronic asthma[65] and is reputed to be a sexual stimulant. For such a gentle oil, it is a surprisingly powerful antiseptic.

Rutaceae

Apart from neroli, orange blossom absolute and petitgrain, oils from the citrus branch of this family are expressed from the peel and referred to as citrus oils; strictly speaking they are essences as the fruits have not been subjected to heat or solvents, therefore they closely resemble the oil in the plant. Such oils should be derived from organically grown fruit – no sprays or pesticides, as these would remain in the expressed oil.

Peel from fruit used for commercial juice production is often distilled, but in fact this process produces inferior oils for aromatherapy as they are usually folded or de-terpenated as well.

Family Properties and Effects   The Rutaceae all produce good digestive oils and most are beneficial to the skin (see each oil).

Caution   Expressed oils contain coumarins (photosensitizers), and should not be used for two hours before going into sunlight or exposure to ultraviolet light (see chapter 6).

Citrus aurantifolia or *C. limetta* – peel (lime) 1.2–2%
Although preferred for aromatherapy, expressed lime oil is difficult to obtain as the aroma of distilled lime is superior (see chapter 5).

Special Properties and Effects   The main attribute of lime oil is its antispasmodic action, but since many oils have this property and you may not know whether or not your oil is expressed, it is preferable to use another oil.

Citrus aurantium var. *amara* – peel (orange bigarade or bitter orange) 0.1–0.4%
Citrus aurantium var. *sinensis* – peel (orange portugal or sweet orange) 0.3–0.5%
The properties of these two expressed oils are very similar, those of sweet orange being milder, making it a useful oil for children. Like most expressed oils, they are both high in terpenes.

Special Properties and Effects   Sweet orange oil is beneficial for maintaining normal facial skin in good condition, whereas bitter orange can help restore an acne skin to normal and is prophylactic against signs of ageing.

Citrus aurantium var. amara – leaves (petitgrain bigarade) 0.5–1%

Not usually taken from the sweet orange tree, petitgrain is a distilled oil and is sometimes referred to as 'poor man's neroli'; it is not as exotic, though a good one possesses some of the neroli qualities. Petitgrain is much higher in esters and slightly lower in alcohols than neroli; both these constituents are therapeutic and without hazard.

Special Properties and Effects   Petitgrain bigarade is an excellent balancer for dry or oily skin – and the nervous system, relieving irritability and promoting sleep.[66]

Citrus aurantium var. *amara* – flowers (neroli bigarade) 0.08–0.1%

More on oils from the flowers of the orange tree can be found in chapter 5. The blossoms of the sweet orange tree (var. *sinensis*) are rarely distilled and neroli bigarade is, in any case, thought to be more therapeutic than neroli portugal.

Special Properties and Effects   Neroli bigarade is the *pièce de résistance* for broken and varicosed veins, acne, ageing and dry skins. It is extremely effective on nervous problems, such as depression and mental fatigue.

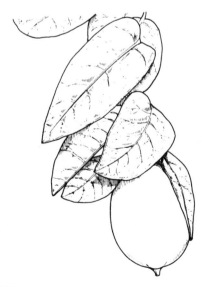

FIGURE 4.6: Bergamot

Citrus bergamia – peel (bergamot) 0.5%

Bergamot trees are vulnerable to root rot, so are usually grown by grafting bergamot cuttings onto stumps of the bitter orange tree;[67] we have seen this being done in Cyprus, for example. The fruit is more oval than round, not quite as oval as a large lemon but with a distinctive point at one end. Farmers with orange groves often grow one bergamot tree for family use; the peel is cooked in a heavy syrup and served with tea in the afternoon – it is delicious! Oil of bergamot is obtained exclusively by expression (the juice is not used) and is extracted when the fruits have almost changed from green to yellow.

Bergamot has a much higher content of esters (around 40 per cent) and alcohols (around 50 per cent) than any other citrus oil (and is lower in terpenes).

Special Properties and Effects   A calming, sedative oil, bergamot is indicated for agitation and insomnia. It also has an antispasmodic action on the stomach, making it useful in cases of gastroenteritis. It is indicated for use on psoriasis and eczema.

Caution   Bergamot is the most phototoxic of the expressed oils (see coumarins in chapter 3).

Citrus limon – peel (lemon) 0.6–0.8%

Lemon oil consists of terpenes (90–95 per cent) and citral (around 5 per cent). A perfume quality oil, originally rich in terpenes, has often had some of these removed, thus effectively raising the citral content. As citral can be irritant to the skin, terpeneless oils should not be used for aromatherapy! (See peppermint above, and chapter 2.)

Special Properties and Effects   Lemon oil is both calming and uplifting and has been used for insomnia.[68] It has more properties than it is given credit for; among these is the fact that it is a good tonic to the liver.

Citrus paradisi – peel (grapefruit) 0.05–0.1%

An oil with the shortest shelf life of the citrus fruit oils, grapefruit oil often has about 0.002 per cent of an antioxidant added to it to lengthen its keeping qualities. In fact, minute amounts of antioxidants are added to most citrus oils for this reason.

Special Properties and Effects   Stimulating and tonic, aperitif and digestive, grapefruit oil also helps to regulate body weight[69] if used regularly. It is an effective air disinfectant.

Citrus reticulata – peel (mandarin, tangerine) 0.7–0.8%
Details of mandarin oil (called tangerine in America) can be found in chapter 5.

Special Properties and Effects   Like bergamot, mandarin is a relaxant, indicated in times of agitation, over-excitement, stress and insomnia. It has weak antispasmodic action, so is good for children's digestive problems. It is also said to be antifungal.[70]

Santalaceae

Santalum album – wood (sandalwood) 4–6.5%
Although it is possible to buy a sandalwood oil distilled from sandalwood trees grown in Australia (*Santalum spicatum* and other species) the aroma is inferior to the Mysore sandalwood produced in the Karnataka region of East India. Those who worry about the exploitation of sandalwood trees may be interested to know that the cutting of trees for distillation is controlled by the government; only trees showing signs of dying are felled, and each is replaced – this has been going on for years. Offcuts and wood chips (from making furniture and decorative boxes) plus the roots are used for distillation. The trees grow in abundance at heights of up to 3,000 feet (just under 1,000 metres) and are parasitic, their roots living on the surrounding undergrowth, eventually killing it.

Containing over 70 per cent of two sesquiterpene alcohols (alpha and beta-santalol), sandalwood is a very therapeutic, yet gentle oil.

Special Properties and Effects   Sandalwood is well known and respected for its balancing effect on the nervous, respiratory and, especially, excretory systems. It is soothing on dry or irritated skin and scalp, including eczema. Considered a sexual tonic, it may be useful for problems related to impotence.

Styracaceae

The trees in this family which interest us do not produce an essential oil, but a gum-resin or oleo-resin called benzoin. The gum is processed into a tincture (by macerating with alcohol), a resin absolute (extracted with hot or cold alcohol), or a resinoid (extracted with a hydrocarbon solvent). See the section on resins in chapter 2 for details of extraction. Benzene, which is often used abroad in the making of a resinoid (it is not allowed in the UK), has the distinct disadvantage to an aromatherapist of being irritating to the skin and toxic by inhalation (there is a permitted level of use). A resin absolute is therefore preferred (see chapter 2).

Styrax tonkinensis – resin (Siam benzoin)
As the gum from this species hardens, it becomes a pale, sometimes translucent, yellowy brown. The oil obtained from it by alcohol extraction has the softest balsamic aroma.

Styrax benzoin – resin (Sumatra benzoin)
This little tree is grown only in Sumatra and the gum exuded is a pale yellowy colour (referred to as the 'almond' grade and being the best quality). When this tree fails to yield any more gum it is scraped to produce an inferior one, which is dark in colour. Sumatra benzoin is more readily available and less expensive than Siam, though generally not of such good quality unless the almond grade is known to have been used.

Special Properties and Effects   Benzoin is well liked for its anticatarrhal and expectorant properties as well as its powerful skin healing effects. It is also a warming oil, making it useful for painful joints and poor circulation.

Umbelliferae, see Apiaceae.

Valerianaceae

Valeriana officinalis – roots (valerian) 0.2–2.0%
Reputedly used as the blueprint for Valium, the well-known sedative drug, valerian is known in the aromatherapy world for its rather pungent aroma. The aroma of the species *V. wallichi* (Indian valerian) is inferior

from a perfumer's point of view, being stronger; the oil is yellowy brown in colour.

European valerian oil is a bluey green, depending on the amount of azulene produced during distillation. As with Roman chamomile, the blue gradually turns greenish if exposed to light, or kept for any length of time. The chemical constituent responsible for the aroma and the therapeutic effects is an ester called bornyl–isovalerate, which develops as the roots are dried. Fresh, well-dried roots yield an aroma which is not too malodorous, but roots kept too long before distilling produce an obnoxious smell and the oil is darker in colour.[71]

Special Properties and Effects   It is used almost exclusively for its powerfully calming effect on the nervous system, thus aiding all conditions related to severe mental stress, e.g. insomnia, agitation, nervous headaches, nervous stomach, palpitations, etc.

Caution   It may not be necessary to use more than one drop of valerian and the addition of petitgrain, orange or mandarin improves the aroma. Overuse for a long period of time may cause lethargy.

N.B. This oil is becoming difficult to obtain and as *Nardostachys jatamansi* (spikenard, or nard), from the same family, is also a powerfully relaxing oil; it can be used in place of valerian.

Verbenaceae

Lippia citriodora or *Aloysia triphylla* – leaves (lemon verbena) 0.07–0.1%
On account of its high price and similarity in aroma to other cheaper lemon-smelling oils, it is extremely difficult to obtain an oil which has not been adulterated with fractions of lemongrass oil.

The labiate *Thymus hiemalis* (common name Spanish verbena) is not a true verbena, though it is often sold as such.

Caution   Because of its high citral content and possible adulteration, lemon verbena may be a skin irritant and should be used with care.

Zingiberaceae

Zingiber officinale – rhizomes (ginger) 3–4.4%

It would be natural to expect ginger oil to have a 'hot' aroma, but unless extracted with carbon dioxide this cannot be, as the molecules responsible for the hotness are too large to come over in distillation, as in black pepper. The oil is taken from freshly ground rhizomes and is richest just under the outer 'skin'.

Special Properties and Effects   The attributes of ginger oil are wide ranging; it is a digestive tonic, relieves toothache, is anticatarrhal, warming to the muscular system (indicating its use for rheumatism) and reputed to be a sexual tonic.

5 *Perplexing Essential Oils – What's In a Name?*

When aromatherapy was first introduced into this country, essential oils were called by their common plant name – rarely by their Latin botanical name. As knowledge on the subject has deepened, the necessity of using the Latin name has become more apparent; it is now extremely important for plant oils to be identified thus.

Sometimes a single common name is given to essential oils from plants which are neither the same genus or species. The oils may contain common factors and the effects be reasonably similar, as in the chamomiles; however, they may be decidedly different, as in the marjorams; one needs to know which essential oil from which group is needed for which purpose. In other instances the oil comes from a plant bearing the same common name and genus, but which is a different species, will contain a constituent not present (or present in a vastly different proportion) in another similarly named genus, e.g. the eucalypti (or eucalypts). In yet other cases, an oil from exactly the same genus **and** species may possess a constituent which is nonexistent in another oil of exactly the same Latin name, e.g. thyme (*Thymus vulgaris*)! This is the most confusing case of all as the specific plant or clone of thyme used (see thyme later in this chapter) affects not only the aroma but more importantly, the effects on the human system.

If an essential oil is labelled and known only by its common name, not only can incorrect use of a powerful, possibly hazardous oil abound but ignorance can result in a friendly oil being labelled as harmful.

I hope it is now becoming clear that there are many facts about certain essential oils which have not been researched sufficiently with specific reference to the Latin name.

It is not possible to cover all oils which may fit into this category, but only to clarify the main oils which can cause confusion.

Basil (Lamiaceae)

Ocimum basilicum var. *album* (European or sweet basil)
Ocimum basilicum var. *basilicum* (exotic basil)

Different varieties of basil come from the same genus and species, therefore have the same basic Latin name.

The question of 'toxicity' arises with respect to basil essential oil on account of its phenolic ether content, made up of methyl chavicol and eugenol. If either is present in high proportions, that sample may need to be used with care. However, there are many varieties of basil, with methyl chavicol contents varying from 3–85 per cent and eugenol from 1–60 per cent. Research shows that an oil tested with a high percentage of methyl chavicol was found not to be toxic[72] and a well-known French authority states that there are no contra-indications known when basil oil is used in the recommended doses.[73] It is also possible that some minor constituents may counteract the effect of the methyl chavicol (this is known as quenching). Tests on humans have produced no irritation at 4 per cent dilution, though mice were irritated at the same strength.[72] It is unfortunate that rodents have been used in the past for research, both from the animals' point of view and the fact that their skin and physiological processes are different from ours, as research has shown that results from animal testing cannot be directly related to humans.[74]

Var. *album*
The oil from this variety is low in phenolic ethers (around 12–18 per cent) and quite high in alcohols (around 50 per cent), making it the oil I prefer to use.

Var. *basilicum*
This variety contains little alcohol, but can have a high percentage of phenolic ethers, which may be rather aggressive with incorrect use.

Camphor (Lauraceae and Dipterocarpaceae)

Cinnamomum camphora (from the wood (camphor); from the leaves (no leaf oil)
Dryobalanops camphora (Borneo camphor)

The subject of camphor oil is a complicated one – 70 pages were written on it by Ernest Guenther, the well-known expert on essential oils.

Cinnamomum camphora

There are two main trees of this same botanical name, the hon-sho (from Japan and China), known as the *true* camphor tree, and the ho-sho (mainly from Formosa), known as the *fragrant* camphor tree.[75]

Both trees produce an oil from the wood (hon-sho containing about 50 per cent camphor and ho-sho, whose camphor (40 per cent) is all in solution and does not crystallize. The leaves of the ho-sho tree yield an oil similar to rosewood (see Rosewood).

True camphor is steam distilled from a crystalline mass which forms under the bark. It is a by-product of the extraction of pure camphor, which can crystallize at normal temperatures, so a coiled condenser cannot be used in the cooling process. It is a lengthy procedure, the oil produced at this stage being called crude camphor, which is always rectified (fractionated) under vacuum to separate out three different grades or fractions - white, brown and blue, which vary in composition greatly with each sample of oil. The one invariably sold to aromatherapists is the white fraction, which can have a significant content of camphor (a ketone) and cineole (an oxide), a total of 30–50 per cent of constituents which constitute a hazard. A coiled condenser can be used for the extraction of ho-sho wood oil as camphor crystals do not separate out of this oil.[75] Ho-sho *wood* oil, from which camphor and linalool (its main constituents) could be isolated, is not used so much now for linalool extraction, as ho *leaf* oil contains a much higher percentage of this precious chemical. However, even this source of linalool is used less and less, as linalool can easily and cheaply be made synthetically.

The leaf oil from the ho-sho tree is principally composed of linalool, an alcohol; it competes in aroma with rosewood oil and presents no hazards (see Rosewood below). High grades of ho leaf oil contain very little camphor and the oil was mainly used for extracting linalool for use in the perfume industry. If a genuine ho leaf oil unaltered in any way could be obtained, it would make an excellent substitute for rosewood oil.

Dryobalanops camphora

Valnet refers not to *Cinnamomum camphora* for aromatherapy use, but to *Dryobalanops camphora* (Borneo camphor) from the plant family Dipterocarpaceae; this tree produces an oil with totally different properties. *D. camphora* also comes from a crystalline mass which forms under the bark, exactly like that of *C. camphora*; however, *D. camphora* contains mainly alcohols and hardly any ketones, making it an essential oil without hazard. It is erroneously referred to as the wood-extracted camphor (easily obtainable) – the perfect reason for using Latin names, *D. camphora* is, unfortunately, not now readily available and Valnet's indications for its use should not be referred to as representing *C. camphora*.

Cedarwood and Juniper (Abietaceae and Cupressaceae)

Cedrus atlantica (Atlas cedarwood)
Cedrus deodora (Himalayan or Deodar cedarwood)
Juniperus procera (East African cedarwood)
Juniperus mexicana (Texas cedarwood)
Juniperus virginiana (Virginian cedarwood)
Juniperus oxycedrus (cade)
Juniperus communis (juniper)
Juniperus sabina (savin)
Thuja occidentalis (white cedar)

There are many more trees than those listed above, with cedarwood as their common name, some belonging to the Abietaceae (or Pinaceae) family, some to the Cupressaceae family. Both these families belong to the Conifer class and need to be mentioned (especially white cedar).

Cedrus atlantica

Growing in the Atlas mountains of North Africa, this conifer closely resembles that of the Lebanon cedar, now a protected species. *Cedrus atlantica* belongs to the pine family and its essential oil is the one most employed by aromatherapists. Comprised mainly of cedrene (50 per cent), a sesquiterpene, and atlantol (30 per cent), an alcohol, cedarwood has many uses.

In France *Cedrus atlantica* is sold only through pharmacists as it is on a restricted list, being cited as neurotoxic and abortive.[76] However, other research shows neither acute toxicity, sensitization or irritation,[77] and although the oil can contain about 20 per cent of atlantone (a ketone), ketones do not always have toxic effects (see chapter 3; also *Thuja occidentalis*) – perhaps this is just such a one.

Cedrus deodora
Also belonging to the pine family, this conifer is closely related to Atlas cedarwood (therefore to the Lebanon cedar) and though its wood is no good for timber, its oil is used in the perfume industry, especially in India, where the tree is grown.

Juniperus procera
Belonging to the Cupressaceae family, this East African tree is the one most used in the production of pencils and wooden boxes. The oil extracted from the waste wood is heavy and viscous, therefore mostly rectified or fractionated for the perfume industry, making it unsuitable for aromatherapy. Large amounts of cedrol and cedranol (alcohols) are isolated from the oil on its arrival in the UK.[78]

Juniperus mexicana
Known as Texas cedarwood this cupressus, grown in Texas, Central America and Mexico, is cut solely for its essential oil (closely resembling that from East Africa). It is also rectified or fractionated as, like the *procera*, it tends to crystallize and become solid. One book gives it as a toxic oil; another says there are no known contra-indications to it. As the main constituents are cedrol (an alcohol) and cedrene (a sesquiterpene) it seems unlikely to be toxic and data available on the whole oil records no acute toxicity or irritation.[79] It is possible that the fractionated oil (see fractionation in chapter 2), or a herbal extract from the plant (see chapter 6) may be toxic.

Juniperus virginiana
The wood from this cupressus is used in the pencil industry and is highly valued, therefore the essential oil is distilled from waste pieces and sawdust. Botanically, the tree is a close relative of East African and Texas 'cedarwoods'. Again, one writer claims there are no known contra-indications to the oil and another that it is an oil to be used with care. Possibly, again, this last opinion applies to the rectified oil or perhaps to

the use of the plant extract rather than the essential oil (see chapter 6). Four research papers give the same non-toxic results as those for *Juniperus mexicana* above.

Juniperus oxycedrus
Cade is the common name of this oil, usually obtained by dry, or 'destructive distillation'.[80] This process yields a crude 'tar', which is rectified before use.

The oil is viscous and dark, staining the skin, and although useful in the treatment of skin and scalp disorders, was withdrawn from use in dermatology several years ago because of the staining, its messiness and possible toxicity.

In 1990, in France, perhaps for the first time *Juniperus oxycedrus* was steam distilled in fractions (see Ylang Ylang below).

Juniperus communis
This is the tree from the cupressus family whose berries, and sometimes twigs and leaves, are distilled to give juniperberry or juniper oil respectively (see chapter 4).

Juniperus sabina
Because of the first part of its Latin name, this bush may be confused with *J. communis* (the same size of bush but with bigger leaves). It is the oil from *J. sabina* which is abortive, not that from *J. communis*. Savin oil was used in the past as an antirheumatic and emmenagogue but, because of its toxicity and irritating effects, has lost much of its former importance.[81] It is still used medicinally in France, but is best not used in complementary aromatherapy.

Thuja occidentalis
Yet another 'cedarwood' from the cupressus family, thuja oil is distilled from the leaves, not the wood, of this tree. This leaf oil needs extreme care in use and is banned from sale in France except through pharmacists. Because of thuja, any oil with the name 'cedarwood' is only available through a pharmacist – the saying 'What's in a name?' means everything where essential oils are concerned!

Do not use in aromatherapy, because of the high thujone (ketone) content, known in this case to be hazardous.

Chamomile (Asteraceae)

Chamaemelum nobile or *Anthemis nobilis* (Roman chamomile)
Chamomilla recutita or *Matricaria chamomilla* (German chamomile)
Ormenis mixta or *Ormenis multicaulis* or *Anthemis mixta* (Moroccan chamomile)

Chamomile flowers contain a colourless compound which decomposes during distillation to produce azulene, changing to a blue colour in the process.

Chamaemelum nobile
This to my mind is the best all-round oil of the three – it is certainly my favourite. Having a less pungent aroma than that of *Chamomilla recutita*, the double, cultivated Roman chamomile flower consists almost entirely of petals and the yellow centre (receptacle) is solid. The flowerheads are used as a medicinal herb and are also distilled to produce an essential oil (high in esters) which varies from a clear bluish-green to greenish-yellow, depending on the amount of azulene produced during distillation. The wild variety of the same Latin name has only one row of petals and is often referred to as Scotch chamomile.[82]

Chamomilla recutita
C. recutita has a single row of fine, narrow petals around its prominent, hollow centre. As the flower matures, the petals bend backwards to reveal the conical shape of the yellow centre. Much more azulene is produced from the flowerheads of this plant during distillation than from *C. nobile*, resulting in a dark blue essential oil with a pungent aroma, which has excellent properties for aiding skin problems.

Ormenis mixta
These plants grow profusely in the wild; 'mixta' means they are wild and a mixture, 'multicaulis' means many-stemmed. In appearance, these plants resemble the wild, single-petalled *Chamaemelum nobile* but the oil is slightly less blue. Steffen Arctander considered *Ormenis mixta* to be no substitute for *C. nobile* in its aroma, due to its lower ester content.[83] Nevertheless, it is higher in alcohols (169 of its constituents have now been identified, the chief ones being santolina alcohol, 38 per cent, and the terpene α-pinene, 15 per cent), and is therefore an interesting oil for

the aromatherapist.[84] Although not recognized as a true chamomile, it appears to emulate many of the effects attributed to its aristocratic relation; the aroma is sometimes as good, depending on the source of the essential oil (occasionally it can be a little sharper). As there has been no research on this oil, the only clues to its effectiveness are through traditional use, as with most essential oils we use! I have found it to be gentle, safe and a good oil to use with others; however it is becoming difficult to find a true *Ormenis mixta* – causing an increase in price.

Clove (Myrtaceae)

Although not exactly a confusing oil, three essential oils can be obtained from the clove tree. As the same Latin name is shared by all three, it is very important when ordering to mention the part of the plant from which you want your oil to come.

Syzygium aromaticum or *Eugenia caryophyllata* (clove)
Bud: This is the best one for aromatherapy, although more expensive than leaf oil. The buds are dried or semi-dried, then comminuted (pulverized) before being water, rather than steam, distilled.

Leaf: This comes from both twigs and leaves, which are collected after the bud and stem harvest and also water distilled. The leaf oil is used by the chemical industry, who extract the phenol eugenol from it; it is not an essential oil in which aromatherapists need take an interest.

Stem: Stems are picked after the buds have been harvested, and are sun dried and *steam* distilled. Clove stem oil is used only by the perfume industry and as a low cost substitute for clove bud oil by the food industry.

All clove oils contain a high percentage of a phenol called eugenol, clove buds containing the lowest.

Eucalyptus (Myrtaceae)

Eucalyptus globulus (blue gum)
Eucalyptus smithii (gully gum)
Eucalyptus radiata (narrow-leaved peppermint)
Eucalyptus citriodora (lemon-scented gum)
Eucalyptus staigeriana (lemon-scented iron bark)

Although there are hundreds of differing types of eucalyptus trees, all belonging to the Myrtaceae family, only a small number of them produce interesting essential oils. Oils from the eucalyptus species with a powerful aroma should be kept away from homoeopathic drugs, as it is said that these are affected by strong smells.

Eucalyptus globulus

The best known eucalyptus tree is kept at a height which makes leaf collection an easy matter. The oil is taken from the fresh or partly dried leaves; although long and thin on a mature tree, the leaves of a young tree are a rounded shape. Australia, once the main producer of eucalyptus oils, has now relinquished this in favour of tea tree oil, subsidized by the government and along with China, the Iberian peninsula is now one of the largest producers of good quality eucalyptus oil.

It is this essential oil with which most aromatherapists are familiar and the essential oil (of which there is an abundance – hence its low cost) is contained deep in the leaves. Although considered a safe oil,[85] it has a high 1,8-cineole content (eucalyptol). Perhaps because of this oxide (though more probably due to the fact that most *E. globus* available is recti-fied, giving it an increased content of 1,8-cineole and a very strong aroma, which could be too reactive for small lungs), it is best to use *E. smithii*, which is a much gentler and safer oil, on small children. If you are currently taking a homoeopathic medicine and wish to use *E. globulus*, do so at a time which leaves a two or three-hour gap between that and the homoeopathic remedy.

Eucalyptus Smithii

This is an extremely gentle oil, despite its high content of 1,8-cineole (eucalyptol), which is an excellent antiviral agent and expectorant, making it a very useful oil for use over the winter period for the whole family. *E. Smithii* is reputed to be energising and uplifting when used in the morning and relaxing and calming when used in the evening.

Eucalyptus radiata

Narrow-leaved peppermint is often used in France in aromatherapy on account of its powerful mucolytic effect. Although it is high in 1,8-cineole, nothing is known to contra-indicate its use.

Eucalyptus citriodora
This species is, at the moment, one of the least used. Although it contains no 1,8-cineole, it has quite a high percentage of citronellal, which is an aldehyde. It should therefore be used in low concentration on people with very sensitive skins.

Eucalyptus staigeriana
A lesser known oil, *E. staigeriana* contains only a small amount of euca-lyptol and has been found to be invaluable for deep-rooted stress, balancing the emotions. On a more symptomatic level, it is analgesic and anti-inflammatory.

Geranium (Geraniaceae)

Pelargonium graveolens or *P.* x *asperum* (geranium, rose ger., ger. rosat)
Pelargonium odoratissimum
Pelargonium roseum

Geranium essential oil (coming only from various species of pelargo-nium) is one of the most valued oils in the perfumery trade, frequently being used to adulterate rose otto and several other oils. Geranium itself is also open to adulteration or cutting, because, like rose, it is an extremely popular aroma for the perfumer.

Some people refer to the geranium oil from the Réunion Isles (some-times called Bourbon geranium) as *Geranium rosat* because of its 'rosy' aroma, which is why geranium oil is often referred to as rose geranium.

However, rose geranium is really a different oil, consisting of either geranium oil distilled over roses, or geranium and rose otto essential oils mixed together.

Pelargonium graveolens
The bulk of geranium oil production comes from this species and a number of countries in the Mediterranean area produce geranium oils from it, varying in quality and aroma. The oil originating from the Bourbon islands was traditionally reputed to be the best; however, Moroccan and Egyptian plants yield a good oil. Geranium oil from China is becoming quite popular although the aroma is not quite so sweet. The price is lower, perhaps because it also gives a higher yield.

Pelargonium odoratissimum
This species of pelargonium was grown for its oil in some southern states of the USA during the first half of the 20th century.

Pelargonium roseum
Thought to be simply a garden name for *P. graveolens*,[86] the geranium of this name was originally grown in Algeria.

Juniper (Cupressaceae)

Juniperus communis (juniperberry oil, juniper oil)
Although, like some 'cedarwood' oils, *J. communis* belongs to the cupressus family, the essential oil is taken from the crushed, dried (or partially dried) berries and not the wood. The confusion here is that sometimes twigs with leaves and berries are distilled, giving rise to **juniper** oil rather than to juni**perberry** oil. Sometimes, berries which have been fermented and distilled in the making of gin are re-distilled to give an inferior oil,[87] so care is needed when purchasing.

Lavender (Lamiaceae)

Lavandula angustifolia (Miller), *L. officinalis* or *L. vera* (true, fine, wild and cultivated)
Lavandula x *intermedia*, sometimes known as *L. hybrida* (lavandin)
Lavandula latifolia (spike lavender)
Lavandula stoechas

The main confusion which exists regarding lavender is the cultivation since the late 1920s of its hybrid 'lavandin' made by crossing true lavender with spike lavender – a different species (at 600 metres the hybrid is produced by nature). Whereas true lavender grows only at high altitudes (above 600 metres – almost 2,000 feet) lavandin grows abundantly and happily on much lower ground (400–600 metres) which makes it easier to cultivate. It is all grown from cuttings (i.e., it is cloned).

Because lavandin is so much less expensive, farmers began to neglect their lavender plants as nobody wanted to pay the necessarily high price; the production of lavender oil has therefore decreased continually as a result.[88] This state of affairs was reached as early as the years of the Second World War.

From late June until the harvest in late July or early August hundreds of fields in Provençe present a wonderful rich bluey purple for the tourists to enjoy – all of them believing they are looking at lavender! In reality, few tourists experience the more pinky purple of true lavender, as the roads up the mountains are too small and winding for coaches. There are places accessible by car where lavender can still be seen and it also grows abundantly on steep stony slopes by the road and on the plateaux which can be reached on foot.

Cloned lavandin plants yield almost twice as much oil as lavender and are much easier to grow. Apart from *L. x intermedia* 'Super', lavandin essential oil does not have the sweetness of lavender, but is strong, and therefore good enough for soaps and soap powders – a major use previously satisfied by the much more expensive lavender oil. It is also a cheap source of linalool, a constituent valuable in the perfume trade.

L. angustifolia (Miller), *L. officinalis* and *L. vera*

The true lavender plant is easily distinguished by its small delicate flower-heads and there are no side shoots from the main stem. Its colour varies from lilac to deep mauve (occasionally white lavender can be found) and it grows best in very dry, stony, limey soil.

This one species (with three names) yields what is known as 'fine' lavender ('vera' means true). The research establishment in Provençe (Laboratoire Plantes Aromatiques) tells me that most lavender oil now produced in France is from the plant *L.angustifolia* Miller, and it is the only true, fine lavender recognized by the French Pharmacopoeia. When lavender is cultivated from the seeds of these plants, 'population' lavender is the result (see also 'thyme' in this chapter). However, when cuttings are taken from the hardiest and strongest plants and these clones are cultivated, the resulting strains are given an additional appendage. At the time of writing, one–sixth of the true lavender produced in France is from 'Maillette' plants.

Lavandula x *intermedia*

Lavandin, which was 'invented' by crossing true lavender and spike lavender, has practically replaced true lavender in the perfume world because of the greater quantity of oil it produces and the lower price it commands. The flower of this hybrid is closer knit and bigger than that of lavender, the shape of one or two varieties (there are several) being like a cone. Lavandin

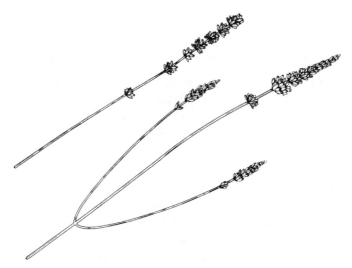

FIGURE 5.1: Fine lavender and lavandin – relative sizes and shapes

is easily recognized by the flower and by the two large side stems (also with flowers) emerging about 20 cm down most of the main stems.

Of the three varieties, 'Super' has the most esters, 'Grosso' produces the most oil but has fewer esters, and 'Abriale' is now little produced due to disease. 'Reydovan' is a strain with fewer esters and more camphor.[89]

Lavandula latifolia

This large plant has close-knit flowerheads with two small side stems, and yields spike lavender oil, the aroma of which is very camphoraceous. The yield is very high, making it an inexpensive oil, and because of this, together with the fact that it will grow at much lower altitudes (thus making farming simpler), this is the plant which was crossed with true lavender (giving lavandin) in the late 1920s in the hope of obtaining an oil with the aroma of lavender and the yield of spike.

Spike lavender is now grown mostly in Spain.

Lavandula stoechas

The essential oil from this species of lavender contains about 70 per cent of ketones, suggesting that it may be an oil aromatherapists need not use – its therapeutic effects can be found in other oils.

Lime (Rutaceae and Tiliaceae)

Citrus aurantifolia or *Citrus limetta* (lime)
Tilia europaea or *Tilia cordata* (lime or linden blossom)

The confusion here exists because when people talk about lime blossom they often omit the word 'blossom' and of course without this word one thinks of the citrus fruit, which is totally different! Both are interesting as far as essential oils are concerned.

Citrus aurantifolia – zest

Lime oil is not, as one would think, obtained predominantly by expression; in fact, very little expressed oil of lime is produced. The distilled oil is more lime-like in aroma and is therefore more useful to the food and perfume industries. Sometimes the whole fruit is distilled, when the resultant distillate separates into three layers. The middle layer is comprised of juice and the top and bottom layers containing the essential oil are then slowly re-distilled to obtain the final essential oil.

Tilia europaea

This beautiful tree belongs to the Tiliaceae family. The harvesting of lime blossom, or linden blossom, as it is also known, is an important industry in the south of France, where the blossoms are collected, dried and packaged as a tea. It can take more lime blossoms even than rose petals to yield one litre of essential oil, so genuine lime blossom oil is not readily available – the cost would be prohibitive! When an oil is offered for sale as lime blossom for less than the cost of rose otto, it cannot be genuine and may be a macerated oil (see chapter 8).

Lime blossom tea is an excellent relaxant, ideal for hyperactive children, is helpful in colds and flu and in reducing blood pressure. As we have two beautiful trees outside our French farmhouse, I drink the tea for its flavour alone, or to relax before going to bed if I have had a stressful day.

Marigold (Asteraceae)

Calendula officinalis (Garden marigold, pot marigold or calendula)
Tagetes glandulifera (French marigold)

Of the two marigolds, only one produces an essential oil.

Calendula officinalis

Essential oil is not obtained from *C. officinalis* commercially, although at one time an absolute was produced in France. It grows almost like a weed in most gardens, the depth of orange in the flowers determining the colour of the macerated oil, which is produced on a commercial scale. Because the healing properties of the flowers are taken into the vegetable oil used in the maceration process, calendula oil provides a useful base for aromatherapy massage, not only for its own merits, but also to enhance the properties of the essential oils added (especially where there is inflammation or any problem concerning the skin – see chapter 8).

Tagetes glandulifera

Tagetes, a powerful essential oil because of the high percentage of ketones present, is distilled from the African marigold and needs to be used with care (see chapter 4).

Marjoram and Oregano (Lamiaceae)

Origanum majorana or *Majorana hortensis* (sweet marjoram, knotted marjoram)
Thymus mastichina (Spanish marjoram, Spanish wild marjoram)
Origanum vulgare (oregano, wild marjoram, garden marjoram)
Thymus capitatus (Spanish oregano)

Essential oils with the common names of both marjoram and oregano come from the labiate family and some, with the common name oregano, come from the verbena family. Even botanists find it difficult to classify the marjorams and oreganos! Because of this, it is extremely important to know the properties and effects of the oil obtained from the plant of the Latin name. Origanum means 'joy of the mountain'.

> 'One of the most confused areas of botanical perfumery nomenclature is that of … marjoram – origanum – thyme. For many decades, outstanding authors and authorities have done their best to straighten out this confusion, but some suppliers continue to mislabel their materials, overlooking all the efforts made to establish correct names.' [90]

Origanum majorana

O. majorana has small 'knots' of white or pink flowers in almost rounded heads and the leaves are a greyish green. The oil from it is a pale yellowy brown colour, deepening with age and the aroma is softer and sweeter than *T. mastichina* (Spanish marjoram).

O. majorana is the essential oil written about in aromatherapy books and the oil which should be purchased if the effects written about it are desired. Unfortunately, the marjoram usually supplied is the less expensive *T. mastichina*, which, as the genus clearly shows, is a thyme and therefore contains different constituents. The major component in Spanish marjoram is that powerful oxide, 1,8-cineole, needing care in use, whereas true marjoram has a significant content of therapeutic and hazard-free alcohols and esters (around 40 per cent of each). This, with its low or non-existent phenol content (0–0.5 per cent) makes it a safe oil for general use.[91] The only reference I can find to do with reproduction is that it is very calming to the oversexed! Neither Lautié and Passebecq, Durrafourd, Valnet nor other French writers mention it in connection with stimulating periods or having an emmenagogic action. Culpeper says that the **plant** 'provokes women's courses' if put up as a pessary, but he is talking about the plant, not essential oil; every therapeutic action of a plant cannot be assumed to apply also to the oil or vice versa (see chapter 6). However, many British writers give *O. majorana* as a menstrual stimulant, myself included, until my French, my general plant knowledge and my chemistry improved and I realized how the mis-understanding may have arisen. One French writer, Philippa Mailhebiau, does say that it works very well (like clary) on young women who are apprehensive about their periods – spasms, pain and anxiety.[92] Yet another gives the same therapeutic effects as the other French writers but gives the phenolic content (thymol and carvacrol) as 80 per cent! He has perhaps used a GLC reading on *Origanum vulgare* by mistake ... all very confusing.

I am certain that *Origanum majorana* is safe to use (in a controlled manner) during pregnancy, but as most suppliers do not use Latin names and therefore may pass on *T. mastichina* (Spanish marjoram) instead of the true marjoram, it is safer to treat all marjorams with care until education on the subject is universal.

Thymus mastichina

This 'impostor', usually labelled as marjoram, grows mainly in the Iberian peninsula, hence 'Spanish' marjoram. It has fewer monoterpenes and alcohols, a few more esters and a very variable content of the oxide, 1,8-cineole (5 up to 80 per cent) if it is 'population' (grown from seed). Any hazards would depend on the cineole content of plants grown from seed or from cuttings (clones) of a known composition.

Origanum vulgare
The common garden herb, *O. vulgare*, often referred to as wild marjoram, is cultivated all over the world more for use in cooking than for its essential oil,[93] which has a high phenol content.

Thymus capitatus
Most oregano essential oil is obtained from *T. capitatus* – which has very powerful antiseptic qualities, due to the phenols, of which it contains a significant amount. It is therefore irritating to the skin and slightly toxic, and should only be used by a well-qualified aromatherapist, if at all.

Melissa (Lamiaceae)

Melissa officinalis (lemon balm or heart's delight)
So little true melissa essential oil is produced that some people think none is available, yet we watch our melissa being distilled every year! The plant, although it grows abundantly, producing the most wonderfully aromatic leaves in profusion, contains very little essential oil. It needs not only a special electronically controlled still and an expert distiller, but if harvested when wet or at the wrong time of day, it can yield no oil at all! As a result the cost is rather higher than distilled rose otto.

The aroma of melissa is easily copied and, apart from lemon verbena and jasmine absolute, it is probably the most adulterated oil found in the perfume industry, which mostly (if not always) mixes its own 'melissa', using various other lemon smelling oils such as lemon, lemongrass and citronella and/or isolated aromatic aldehydes, together perhaps with synthetic components.[94] The therapeutic effects of this oil are not those of true melissa, but a mixture of the properties of those oils in the mix, which are uplifting and refreshing.

True melissa is a wonderful oil for women and a tea made from the leaves and drunk daily is said to promote a long, healthy life (most of the melissa grown in France is dried to make melissa tea).

Orange (Rutaceae)

Citrus aurantium var. *amara* (bitter orange or Seville orange)
Citrus aurantium var. *sinensis* and var. *dulcis* (sweet orange)
Citrus reticulata or *C. madurensis* or *C. nobilis* (mandarin or tangerine)

A whole book could be written on the orange tree and its essential oils. When ordering, the Latin name should be given, plus the part of the plant from which the oil comes and, for flower oils, it is essential to state whether distilled or absolute oil is required. Three different oils (from peel, leaf and flower) are produced from two varieties of one species.

Citrus aurantium var. *amara*

Oils from the bitter orange tree are known as 'bigarade' oils; neroli bigarade is distilled oil from the blossoms (orange blossom bigarade is an absolute); petitgrain bigarade is distilled from the leaves and orange bigarade is obtained by expression from the fruit peel.

Neroli bigarade oil has an exquisite aroma and is around 30 times the price of leaf and fruit oils, the petals having far fewer oil glands per kilo of plant material. I was interested to see both blossoms and fruit present on the tree at the same time. Neroli is often confused with the absolute, which is called 'orange blossom' oil and has a totally different aroma, viscosity and colour.

Citrus aurantium var. *sinensis*

Oils from the sweet orange tree are known as 'portugal' oils and their aroma is generally lighter (the leaves are not usually distilled).

Neroli portugal oil is considered to be of a lesser quality than neroli bigarade and is more often used to adulterate neroli bigarade than as an oil in its own right.

Orange portugal, from the peel and known as sweet orange, is similar in characteristics to orange bigarade and, having a 'weaker' effect, is suitable for use on children, old people and pregnant women. As with lime, a purely expressed oil is difficult to obtain, as the juice industry tend to distil the oranges after extracting the juice. The sheer size of this industry in America causes a glut of orange oil. The distilled oil often has antioxidant added, as it tends to oxidize far more quickly than the expressed oil.[95] Cyprus produces a superior expressed oil, with the best keeping qualities.

Citrus reticulata

Many people believe mandarin and tangerine oils differ from each other; in fact nowadays the two names refer to the same oil. Tangerine is the name used in America, and both tangerine and mandarin oil may be traded as mandarin. Some botanists say the trees are from different varieties of *Citrus reticulata* and others say they both come from *Citrus madurensis*. Oil from tangerine trees was originally different from mandarin and used to be nearer to bitter orange than to mandarin; however, as perfumers found it a rather 'dilute' aroma without much character, growers developed the tangerine tree to give the characteristics of the mandarin. In the past, tangerines were always larger than mandarins – now it is very difficult to distinguish between the two.

Peppermint (Lamiaceae)

Mentha arvensis (cornmint)
Mentha x *piperita* (Mitcham mint)

Mentha arvensis

In America, if the oil from this plant is used, it has to be referred to as 'cornmint' or simply mint. The plant originated in Japan and is not a true peppermint.[96] However, its cheapness makes it a popular oil in the perfume industry and because it contains a high percentage of menthol (often up to 80 per cent) some of this can be removed by freezing (menthol crystallizes at low temperature) and used in the pharmaceutical industry. The remaining oil is often sold as peppermint oil and is also often adulterated to increase the pepperminty aroma. The removal of the menthol obviously increases the percentage of menthone in cornmint oil; in a de-mentholized oil menthone is present in amounts of up to 26 per cent.

It has been customary to use *Mentha arvensis*, known all over the world (except the USA) as 'peppermint oil' and the lower cost of the de-mentholized oil is very tempting.[97] The Japanese *Mentha arvensis* can contain 20–30 per cent pulegone; this obviously makes it an oil preferably not used during the early stages of pregnancy and possibly accounts for some people believing peppermint generally to be abortive. Again we see the importance of using Latin names.

This oil is not suitable for children under three and should be used with care – or not at all, unless you can guarantee an unadulterated oil.

Mentha x *piperita*

It is generally agreed that this plant is a hybrid from *Mentha spicata* (spearmint) and *Mentha aquatica* (water mint). There are many varieties of *Mentha* x *piperita* and the best is of English origin, namely, *Mentha* x *piperita* var. *officinalis, forma rubescens camus*, a rather long name for Mitcham mint, the dark green mint with a purplish stem. Mitcham peppermint plants have been exported all over the world; that grown in England commands a higher price.

When the stem is green, *pallascens* (becoming paler) is substituted for *rubescens* (reddening) in the name.[98]

The essential oil from this plant is a true peppermint and is the only one which, in America, is allowed to be called by that name. Its major ketone content (menthone) varies from 15–30 per cent depending on the country of origin, its menthol content being usually around 55 per cent. When an oil is rectified or folded, the menthone content is proportionately increased and the resulting oil is always colourless. A good peppermint oil will have a slight colour, as do most untreated oils.

Pine (Abietaceae)

Pinus mugo, var. *pumilio* (mountain or dwarf pine)
Pinus palustris (pitch pine)
Pinus sylvestris (Scots pine)

Steffen Arctander considers the pines to be very open to adulteration and considers *Pinus palustris* to give the only 'true' pine oil, although it is rarely available without adulteration and it is not suitable for aromatherapy.

Pinus mugo, var. *pumilio*

There seems to be a slight controversy regarding this oil, one writer saying it has no use in aromatherapy and another giving a long list of its properties, with no contra-indications.[99]

Pinus palustris

It is from this species that turpentine oil is obtained, the resin occurring naturally in the wood, and it is double distilled to obtain it. Turpentine is not an oil which aromatherapists use.

Pinus sylvestris
This is the species that is the best known and most used in aromatherapy (see chapter 4).

Rosewood (Lauraceae and Convolvulaceae)

Aniba rosaeodora – wood (rosewood, bois de rose)
Cinnamomum camphora – leaf (Ho leaf oil)

Aniba rosaeodora
Aniba rosaeodora from the Lauraceae family is felled mainly for its wood. The essential oil from Cayenne in French Guiana was always hailed as having the best aroma, but very little is now produced there, Peru and the northern areas of Brazil being responsible for most of the oil produced.

Containing a very high percentage of fine quality linalool (around 90 per cent) the oil was used in the past mainly to isolate this component for the standardization of other essential oils. Perhaps it is fortunate that nowadays this source has strong competition from synthetic linalool!

In Brazil the tree was an endangered species until replacement planting began, but this has not worked, and the new trees are unable to grow healthily because of the condition of the soil, due to forest destruction.[100] Also, many people still do not like to see the essential oil used, for environmental reasons. For such people there is a solution – apart from ho leaf oil. *Convolvulus scoparius*, grown in the Canary Islands and from a totally different family, the Convolvulaceae, has as one of its common names 'rosewood'. Usually referred to as rhodium wood oil, the aroma is similar to that of *A. rosaeodora* – hence no doubt the acquisition of the name 'rosewood'. *Convolvulus scoparius* generally appears on the market not as the true oil, but as a blend, from mixing together geranium or palmarosa oil with a touch of sandalwood.[101] For those who feel strongly about the rainforests (even with replacement planting), why not experiment with the oils mentioned so that you can enjoy a rosewood aroma? I am doing a blend myself called 'rosewood mix' (or 'caring man's rosewood'!) until I can guarantee a genuine and whole ho leaf oil or *C. scoparius* essential oil.

The mixed oil still has therapeutic properties (those of the individual oils used) and if you make a list of these you will be surprised at some of the similarities with the true oil, including the uplifting and bactericidal properties.

A blend of geranium and sandalwood would certainly be effective on several skin conditions; however, if you wish to have true rosewood, you need to purchase your oil with care, and not from a perfume source.

Cinnamomum camphora (from the leaves)
Distilled ho leaf oil, as it is called, is taken from the variety of *C. camphora* known as the ho-sho tree. The aroma is similar to bois de rose oil from Brazil *(Aniba rosaeodora)* and it is sometimes sold as such – both have a high linalool content.[102] A high grade ho leaf oil should contain very little camphor and would have interesting properties for the aromatherapist, were it possible to ensure that it was unadulterated (see chapter 4).

Thyme (Labiateae or Lamiaceae)

Thymus vulgaris, ct. carvacrol (red thyme)
Thymus vulgaris, ct. thymol (red thyme)
Thymus vulgaris, ct. geraniol (sweet thyme)
Thymus vulgaris, ct. linalool (sweet thyme)
Thymus vulgaris, ct. thujanol-4 (sweet thyme)
Thymus vulgaris, ct. alpha-terpineol (sweet thyme)

Here we have a plant from the labiate family which produces, from a single species, at least six different essential oils. How is this possible? No one knows! The plants look identical, but when growing in the wild the chemical constituents vary considerably from plant to plant, as do also the aromas. This is easy to prove while on a mountain walk. We often squeeze identical looking thyme plants and savour the vastly differing aromas. Because of this variation the 'types' of thyme are called chemotypes or occasionally chemovars. When the *seeds* from one chemotype are used to produce new plants, there is no guarantee that they will be the same chemotype as the parent plant, so when thyme oil is distilled from these, as with wild thyme plant seeds, the resulting oil is called 'population' thyme; it contains a mixture of all the components that are possible from the different chemotypes and should therefore be a good 'average' thyme oil for aromatherapy.

However, when it is more important to ensure exclusively one particular component, how is this guaranteed? It can be done! A plant is tested for its constituents and when cuttings are taken and grown from that particular plant, the same chemotype will develop. In other words they are cloned, although the thujanol clone does not grow well.

Although all six oils are different, we can, to simplify matters, split them into two groups, using the name of the chemical family constituent most predominant.

Thymes containing phenols (phenolic thymes, often known as red thymes). These two are high in phenols, which makes them extremely powerful antiseptics. However, they can be aggressive and also skin irritants if used in a concentrated form, therefore both should be used with care and are best left in the hands of qualified therapists.

Thymes containing alcohols (usually known as sweet thymes). The predominant component in each of these four oils is an alcohol. Many of the properties of these sweet thymes overlap; all are antibacterial, immunostimulant, a tonic to the nervous system and all help cystitis, arthritis, sinusitis and skin problems such as eczema. Alcohols are gentle and kind, so all of these thymes can be used safely at any time, even on children.[103]

I am sure you can now understand why thyme is an oil where it is important to ask either for the specific chemotype or stipulate 'red' or 'sweet'.

There are many other species of thyme, among them are *Thymus mastichina* ('marjoram') and *Thymus capitatus* ('oregano'), discussed under 'marjoram' above. *Thymus serpyllum*, wild thyme, which grows profusely in the wild in the hills and mountains of southern France, is used mainly in the pharmaceutical and cosmetic industry and *Thymus citriodora*, the lemon-scented thyme, provides a different colour and flavour for the herb garden.

Note: Only the phenolic thymes need to be used with care.

Ylang Ylang

Cananga odorata
There is no botanical confusion with this oil, but its distillation is so complex, and so open to adulteration, that it needs to be explained.

The flowers of *Cananga odorata* are distilled over a period of up to 24 hours, usually being 'interrupted' to keep the smallest molecules, which come off first, separate from the rest. This is because this first fraction of the oil (sometimes taken as two separate fractions) has the sweetest and most floral aroma and is therefore of greatest value to the perfumer. It is called 'ylang ylang extra'; if there are two fractions the second is called 'ylang ylang superior' and these are the most expensive of the ylang ylang oils. The distillation process is then continued, interrupted once more, and the next group of essential oil molecules to arrive at the end of the collecting vessel is named 'ylang ylang 1' which is a different quality oil. It is up to the distiller when to stop the distillation for the 'extra' quality and as it is a subjective judgement the quality of this oil is quite variable.[104] The process of distillation with interruption is carried out twice more, yielding 'ylang ylang 2' and 'ylang ylang 3'; the whole process can take up to 24 hours.

In actual fact, about 10 fractions are taken; one and two become extra or are kept separate (named 'extra' and 'superior'), fractions three, four and five may become grade 1; fractions six and seven become grade 2; and eight, nine and ten become grade 3. The fractions are evaluated into the 4 or 5 grades by the distiller's personal feelings on aroma. The solubility in alcohol deteriorates towards the second and third grade, which may be why the oil is fractionated, although the third quality is used extensively in perfumery.

The chemist will often judge the oil according to its ester content, but this figure is unfortunately an easy one to arrange by the addition of synthetic esters.[105]

All fractions are open to cheating or adulteration; 'extra' is mostly adulterated with 'no 1' and sometimes with grades 2 and 3 – the lowest quality. Vanillin, isolated components from other, cheaper oils, or even synthetic components are often added. Grade 2 is not a popular oil on its own, so is reserved for 'cutting' or adulterating ylang ylang extra and grade 1. The complete oil, containing the components from all four fractions, is called 'ylang ylang complete', but sadly this is the most abused of all the ylang ylangs as it does not always contain the top fraction. If one could obtain a true complete oil, this theoretically should be the best for aromatherapy as it is not fractionated[106] but no-one seems sure about its quality or 'wholeness'. Until we can go to the Comores or Nossi-Be ourselves and get to know one of the farmers there, I shall continue to have reservations about this popular oil. The procuring of ylang ylang essential oil is a minefield – and anyone's guess!

6 *Safety of Essential Oils*

Introduction

'Aromatherapy' is defined as the **controlled** use of essential oils in a positive way to maintain good health and revitalize the body, mind and spirit.

'Essential oils' are defined thus: 'Essential oils are the exclusive product of the extraction of the volatile aromatic principles contained in the substances of which they bear the name' (Geneva conference). For therapeutic aromatherapy, I prefer a more precise definition, which excludes all concretes, absolutes, resinoids and gums, so that the term essential oil embraces only the volatile distilled oils plus essences expressed from citrus fruits.

The epithet 'essential' was first applied to plant volatile oils to describe them as being like an essence (from 'quintessentia') – not in the sense that they were indispensable to the plant. They are, in fact, secondary metabolites. This may sound a little disappointing, but it may be some comfort to reflect that the word 'oil' is also a misnomer.

Essential oils are not perfect, but they are useful practical tools which we can use in a caring situation with success and delight.

Herbalism and Aromatherapy

Herbalism, using plants and their extracts (very occasionally essential oils – not necessarily the same ones as used in aromatherapy) has been practised for centuries. When scientific medicine was introduced, herbalism waned for a while, until the revival of natural aids to good health.

Although inevitably there are people who attend short non-qualifying courses on herbalism, and set up in practice (as with many complementary therapies, unfortunately), qualifying to be a medical herbalist is normally a four-year training, involving in-depth studies of plants, together with their beneficial, and hazardous, properties and effects. Aromatherapy, on the other hand, was first introduced as a post-graduate course for beauty therapists – an extra, to enhance the qualifications already held (which did not include medical or diagnostic knowledge). The average length of a course was only four days, which meant there was little chance to learn much about essential oils, as most of the time was spent learning a specialized massage.

This would not have been important had aromatherapy remained exclusively for beauty therapists; all oils used during the first decade of the therapy being practised (with massage as the only method of use) were already blended and diluted in vegetable oil – there was no responsibility on the part of the therapist for selecting individual essential oils.

However, when complementary massage therapists, acupuncturists, etc. and caring lay people (willing first to qualify in massage, anatomy and physiology) expressed an interest in aromatherapy, it was inevitable that essential oils were individually and holistically selected. When this happened, those teaching aromatherapy realized that much more essential oil theory was required and bona fide courses significantly increased in length as a result, much of the extra information being taken at that time from herbal text books such as Culpeper and Mrs Grieve etc. It will take a few years to sort out any incorrect suppositions now recorded in aromatherapy books.

To provide knowledge on properties and effects of *plants* (and essential oils, where mentioned) books like the above are ideal sources; however, the properties and effects of a plant are not always the same as those of its essential oil. Dominique Verdet, a doctor who, after qualifying, studied phytotherapy for three years at Bobigny university, says:

'We must make the point that many oils have very different therapeutic indications from the plants from which they came. This is contrary sometimes to Dr Valnet's indications. For example, the eucalyptus oil is an expectorant. The garlic clove is hypotensive through its juice – the oil stimulates bleeding and prevents clotting.

More and more we discover new qualities of the plant and new qualities of the essential oil, and we find it does not always correspond. In former times they thought both had the same therapeutic qualities.'[107]

When a herbal remedy specifies use of a particular extract of the plant (tisanes and extracts with alcohol etc.), the resulting constituents contain molecules which are too large to come over in distillation. Just as resins and absolutes are different chemically from an essential oil (see chapter 2), herbal extracts are also chemically different from an essential oil.

Distilled oils: contain only volatile molecules, very limited in size (see chapter 3).

Expressed oils: contain molecules of all sizes (including large ones).

Absolutes: contain molecules of all sizes, but only those soluble in both the solvent used and alcohol; not necessarily all, or only, the volatile ones.

Resinoids: contain molecules of all sizes, but only those soluble in the particular solvent used for the extraction process; not necessarily all the volatile ones.

Macerated oils: contain molecules of all sizes which are soluble in vegetable oil; not necessarily all the volatile ones.

Plant extracts: contain all molecules which are soluble in the liquid being used for the extraction process; not necessarily all the volatile ones.

Much information has been recorded on the therapeutic qualities of herbs – less on essential oils. Although some therapeutic effects overlap, the different chemical structures dictate that not only benefits must vary, but also any toxicity.

There is a long list of plants (and essential oils) used in medical herbalism and perfumery which are exceedingly toxic; as are many of the plants used in homoeopathy. Aromatherapists without training in herbal medicine do not utilize any of these. The 'toxicity' of those which *are* used has been researched mainly by the fragrance industry for application on the skin and by a few universities from different parts of the world for internal use, mainly using animal testing, which is not conclusive for humans.[74]

On the skin, aromatherapists normally use dilutions around 1–3 per cent and, so long as people are aware of the few hazards there are (and do not misuse the oils), there should be very little danger.

Synergy

We know the properties and effects of each group of chemicals; what we do not know yet is how these effects may change in the overall special combination of chemical constituents in each plant. There is certainly more to essential oils than meets the eye!

It has been proved by Valnet that the bactericidal effect of a mix of oils is greater than the sum total of the individual oils. There is no scientific explanation for this – nor for many of the apparent phenomena of essential oils. Why, for example, is one oil with a very low percentage of a toxic component credited with a contra-indication, when another, having an equal or higher percentage of that same component, has been found to be completely safe?

Take, for example, *Eucalyptus globulus* and *E. smithii* – each containing around 60–70 per cent of the oxide, 1,8-cineole, yet *E. smithii* is not contra-indicated for use on young children as is *E. globulus*![108] This apparent contradiction (and many others) goes to show how complex is the study of essential oils and the present state of knowledge of aromatherapy.

Also, cinnamic aldehyde, when isolated from whole cinnamon bark oil, is a severe skin irritant, yet the whole oil, in 8 per cent dilution, does not appear to be the irritant expected on humans (unless used neat), though it is on mice and rabbits, whose skin is different (see Synthetic Oils in chapter 2) – I wish more research was founded on human experiences.

The following quotation on sensitization is a further example:

> 'In the course of maximization testing in human subjects, three instances arose in which an individual aldehyde occurring widely in nature proved to be a skin sensitizer. However, the essential oil in which the aldehyde occurred naturally did not induce sensitization reactions, although the aldehyde was present in concentrations as high as 85 per cent. It appears now to be a consistent finding that these aldehydes, although producing sensitization reactions when applied alone, produce

no sensitization reactions in selected simple mixtures with other compounds."[9]

D. L. J. Opdyke, 1976

There has not been sufficient research carried out yet to have discovered either facts like the above, or every possible health problem each essential oil is capable of helping. Serious writers on aromatherapy may have discovered a situation where an oil will help something no-one has yet mentioned – I know this has been true for me over the years. I always tell people who do not possess the essential oil indicated for their problem to try one they do have and they may be lucky! One of our teachers in the USA had to return home from work once because of a high temperature and the onset of what she thought was flu. She had left work without her essential oils and could find only lemongrass at home; although not indicated for flu, she used it in the shower, in a vaporizer and on a tissue while in bed and she could not believe how well she felt the next morning.

N.B. Lemongrass contains around 70 per cent citral – whose irritant effect can be quenched by mixing 50/50 with an oil whose d-limonene content is equal to or higher than the aldehyde content in the lemongrass. Two citrus oils containing around 90 per cent of dextro-limonene are sweet orange and grapefruit, making them excellent oils to use[109] (see chapter 2).

Safety

Before anything was published regarding the use of certain oils in pregnancy, women, pregnant or not, were using any essential oil they wished in the sensible and rational methods and dilutions advocated in aromatherapy books (their only source of knowledge!) without any recorded ill effects, even from those who were pregnant. Remember, aromatherapy is the *controlled* use of essential oils; when used thus there are no more hazards than with many other things we use daily (e.g. alcohol, aspirins, bleach, etc.) – and they are a lot less dangerous than many prescribed drugs taken nowadays regularly. A great number of people in hospital are there because of the side effects of the drugs they have been given – not only because of the original condition. There have been more deaths as a result of the action of medical drugs (and aspirins, alcohol and even potatoes!) than there have been people even slightly ill as a result of

Key to Cautions

N	Not Proven
r	Rare
u	Unlikely
C	Care till researched
*	Not normally sold to aromatherapists
**	No hazards with complete oil

■ High %

◨ Medium %

◩ Low %

◪ V. Low %

N.B.

Clary, melissa, myrrh and rose otto are hormone balancing oils and considered safe during pregnancy.

Oil Name	Latin Name
Aniseed	*Pimpinella anisum*
Angelica Root	*Angelica archangelica*
Basil (exotic)	*Ocimum basilicum v. basilicum*
Bergamot	*Citrus aurantium v. bergamia*
Camphor	*Cinnamomum camphora*
Cinnamon Bark	*Cinnamomum zeylanicum*
Clove Bud	*Syzygium aromaticum*
Clove Leaf	*Syzygium aromaticum*
Eucalyptus	*Eucalyptus globulus*
Fennel	*Foeniculum vulgare v. dulce*
Grapefruit	*Citrus paradisi*
Hyssop	*Hyssopus officinalis*
Juniper* (savin)	*Juniperus sabina* (not *communis*)
Lemon	*Citrus limon*
Lemongrass	*Cymbopogon citratus*
Marjoram, Spanish	*Thymus mastichina*
Marjoram, sweet	*Origanum majorana*
Melissa, True	*Melissa officinalis*
Melissa Mixture	
Nutmeg	*Myristica fragrans*
Origanum	*Origanum vulgare*
Parsley Seed	*Petroselinum crispum*
Peppermint**	*Mentha x piperita*
Pennyroyal*	*Mentha pulegium*
Rose Absolute	*Rosa damascena*
Rosemary (verbenone clone)	*Rosmarinus officinalis*
Sage	*Salvia officinalis*
Savory	*Satureia hortensis*
Tagetes	*Tagetes glandulifera*
Thyme, phenolic	*Thymus vulgaris*

Principal Active Chemicals	%	Skin Irritant	Neurotoxic	Phototoxic	Skin Sensitizer	Abortive	Pregnancy, 0–5 months	Whole Term Pregnancy	Babies
Phenolic ether (anethole)		?			?		X	X	X
Furocoumarins				X					
Phenolic ether (methyl chavicol)		r	C			u	N		C
Furocoumarins				X					
Oxide (1,8-cineole), Ketone (camphone)		X				X	X	X	X
Aldehyde (cinnamaldehyde)		r			X				X
Phenol (eugenol)		?			?				X
Phenol (eugenol)		X			X				X
Oxide (1,8-cineole)		r							X
Phenolic ether (anethole)							X	X	X
Furocoumarins				X					
Ketone (pinocamphone)		X				X	X	X	X
Podophyllotoxine[3]	?	X				X	X	X	X
Furocoumarins				X					
Aldehydes (citral)		X			?				X
Oxide (1,8-cineole)						N	C		X
Phenolic ether (methyl chavicol) - v. low						u			
Aldehyde (citral)		X				u			
Furocoumarins	?	X?		X	X?				
Phenolic ether (myristicin)							X	X	X
Phenols (carvacrol, thymol)		X							X
Phenolic ether (apiole)							X	X	X
Ketone (menthone)		X							X
Ketone (pulegone)			X			X	X	X	X
Solvent extracted		?					N		
Ketone (verbenone)							?		
Ketone (thujone)			X?		r	N	X		X
Phenol (carvacrol)		X							X
Ketone (tagetone)			X			X	X	X	X
Phenols (carvacrol, thymol)		X							X

using essential oils, which 99.9 per cent of the people interested in aromatherapy are using in *extremely* low quantities. Far be it from me not to agree that the *potential* hazards of some of the oils must be given – this is a wise precaution – but in perspective, please. I am certainly not advocating free use of essential oils (even if of good quality) by untrained people.

It seems that some of what has been written on the toxicity of essential oils has been either out of context, without any explanation or reasoning, or greatly exaggerated.

The aim of this chapter is to help allay unnecessary fears, whilst at the same time increasing awareness of the *potential* hazards of essential oils if **misused, abused** or **used in an inappropriate way** (see hospital examples on pages 140–1).

Let us talk first about essential oils which are freely available and yet possess constituents labelled as 'toxic'; oils such as hyssop, sage, nutmeg, thyme and several others, each of which is safe when used properly and **with knowledge**; they certainly should not be available freely to the general public from sources not having a herbalist or aromatherapist on hand to give advice. It is mainly due to the fact that essential oils have been marketed by people without full knowledge of the chemical components and their possible effects, plus lack of full content information on labels, that there exists the possibility of danger with respect to the use of essential oils. Also, some people begin giving aromatherapy workshops after completing only a weekend course (where no mention has been made of any contra-indications to the use of essential oils containing possibly hazardous components).

Essential oils most likely to create a problem are those containing aldehydes, ketones and phenols (including phenolic ethers); therefore understanding and knowledge about the chemistry of essential oils is important (chapter 3). Reputable firms should not offer oils which may present hazards in untrained hands for sale in shops where there is neither an aromatherapist in attendance nor an assistant who has had some training on the oils he or she is selling.

However, now that the seed of doubt has been sown concerning the safety of essential oils, some people may *anticipate* certain reactions (and perhaps even experience them due to a psychological response!), so therapists need to be sure of their facts when asked about essential oils, particularly for specific health conditions. They should be especially aware of the few essential oils presenting possible skin hazards, as this is the area in which they are mostly working.

Vague Information

Up until the late 1980s all essential oils had been used by aromatherapists at any time for any condition and had appeared in books without any reservations. As more information became available, it became known that certain essential oils were hazardous – but not generally why or how. The hows and whys are very important because at that time no dosages were mentioned and the differences between herbs and essential oils was not made clear.

As a result, everyone in the aromatherapy training field was alarmed and lists were made of plant oils 'never to be used in aromatherapy'. Half the oils on these lists are neither taught in schools nor even known by most aromatherapists. They are no doubt readily available to a perfumer or a pharmacist, but neither of these is an aromatherapist. It makes sense that those particular oils should never be made available to the public, but 'never to be used' implies that they are freely available (which they are not) and that they are poisonous – whatever the dose. Poisonous substances are frequently used in the right hands to promote health: it is the dose which is so important (the dilution used), together with the qualifications of the person handling them – knowledge is the important criterion.

To quote Paracelsus – 'All is poison; nothing is poison.'

I am not very fond of the word toxic – it sounds as if it must be injurious in any circumstance (whatever the dose, whatever the method of use), but such is not the case. I prefer to use the word powerful, because even the 'forbidden' oils are beneficial to the health *when used in the correct dilution*, in the right hands and in the right circumstances. If statements regarding the power of certain oils had been accompanied by explanations as to *why* they should be treated with respect and how they need to be used, all the ensuing alarm could have been avoided.

Bottling and Labelling

Even more important, if essential oils were correctly bottled and labelled, most of the few cases with adverse results could have been avoided. For example, in my opinion, integral drop dispensers should only (and always) be fitted in bottles containing 100 per cent essential oil. Bottles containing mainly vegetable oil (or/and alcohol) should not have a drop dispenser – it may confuse the buyer. The label should state clearly what is inside and if diluted, the diluent and the strength should be given, e.g. 1½ per cent, 3 per cent, or whatever. There are several reasons for this:

- The buyer can use diluted oil straight from the bottle on the skin quite safely (making a dropper unnecessary – and slow). Essential oils need to be diluted for use on the skin and even if swallowed, no real harm would be experienced from diluted oils. On the other hand, ready diluted oils are not effective used by the drop in inhalations or the bath, so a drop dispenser is both unnecessary *and* gives the wrong impression of the strength.
- Should the same buyer purchase next time the same sized bottle of the same named plant oil (but be unaware that it contains 100 per cent essential oil) he or she may assume it can be used in the same way as the diluted oil mentioned above.
- Undiluted essential oils are best for inhalation and can be added to carriers for a variety of other uses (see chapter 7). With a drop dispenser, only one drop can escape at a time, and should any be swallowed accidentally, the extreme strength of the taste effectively prevents more from being taken. The pipette type of dropper is *not* safe, as the whole contents are accessible to a child on removal of the cap. One or two drops may make a child cry, but 5–7 ml would have more serious consequences.

Unclear labelling and incorrect bottling procedures can cause confusion to the untrained customer and is much more likely to lead to incorrect use and therefore adverse results.

CASE EXAMPLE

A woman once bought 10 ml of 'oil of peppermint' for indigestion and was told by the shop assistant that rather than massaging it on her abdomen she could swallow a teaspoonful, and relief would be almost immediate. The assistant was trained in how that particular brand name of diluted oils could be used and it turned out that the customer was more than satisfied with the results. However, she next had need of peppermint oil when on holiday, and was unable to locate that particular brand. She purchased some 'peppermint essential oil' without asking how to use it (thinking she already knew) and it was only when taking the spoon up to her mouth that she became aware of the very powerful aroma. Touching it with her tongue, she realized something was wrong, and took it back to the shop, where she learned that this shop only sold neat essential oils and was then advised on how to use these. Both had dropper inserts.

Helpful or Hazardous?

An essential oil can affect a system of the body in different ways. For instance, juniper is stimulating to the kidneys, helping them to perform well if they are sluggish; however, if the kidneys are already overworking, that same oil, incorrectly used, would *over*stimulate them, producing a so-called 'toxic' effect.

Similarly, a few oils stimulate the menstrual flow – useful for someone who has scanty or rare periods, but not advised for someone newly pregnant, whose last wish is to stimulate the onset of a period. But we are talking again of overuse and overdose! These powerful oils only overstimulate if taken in ridiculously high doses *internally* or used in high concentrations for a very long period of time. No-one, except those deliberately trying to promote an abortion or commit suicide would, under normal circumstances, want (or be able) to swallow sufficient oil to be detrimental to the health. (In any case, 10–30 **ml** would be required to be ingested over a very short period of time.)[110]

A misunderstanding often arises between oils which stimulate menstruation and those which help to regulate and balance the hormonal system. The latter oils do not stimulate the menstrual flow, but balance the hormones if the lack of periods is due to hormonal imbalance.[111] Such oils need not necessarily be contra-indicated for use during pregnancy and to be sure, it is best to seek the advice of a professional therapist.

When essential oils are recommended internally by suitably qualified medical or aromatherapy (aromatologist) practitioners the amounts are usually minute: one to three drops, once to three times a day, for a limited period of time (like antibiotics). Essential oils should never be ingested without expert advice, not because the amounts above are dangerous, but because an oil may be contra-indicated for a particular condition – or, due to the particular chemical composition, it is important to know the length of time for which it may be used safely. Especially important for ingestion is the quality of the essential oils being used (see chapter 2).

It is now well accepted by reputable schools, aromatherapy associations and trading houses that essential oils are not for internal use by the layperson . . . so let us talk now about powerful oils with regard to their use externally.

Effects of Essential Oils on the Skin

It has been proved that essential oils can cross the epidermis and thereafter enter the body fluids. However, it has also been shown that the quantity absorbed by the skin is far less than that taken in by ingestion,[112] when every drop finds its way into the body. The main pathways used in aromatherapy for the penetration of essential oils are inhalation and the skin, and the advised proportions are already minimal, usually 6–8 drops for inhalation and baths and 30–60 drops in 100 ml (i.e. 1½–3 per cent for application to the skin). Only a small part of this actually penetrates the body, which means that, when used in the recommended strength, essential oils do not normally present a hazard to the internal organs.

Nevertheless, there are a few oils which, because of their aldehyde, phenol or coumarin content, may irritate the skin or present a problem if used just before going into the sunshine, or act as a sensitizer on some people (see Table 4 on pages 126–127).

Skin Irritation

There are a few oils which, even on a non-sensitive person, may cause irritation on the skin when used neat or in high concentration. The worst offenders are those high in phenols or aldehydes, for example, lemongrass (see N.B. on page 125), dwarf pine, origanum, savory and red thyme (those containing carvacrol and thymol). However, in the dilutions mentioned above, these oils are safe (see synergy on page 124).

If using 2 per cent of a synergistic mix of two, three or four oils in a base, the percentage of each oil present will be less than 1 per cent; if this mix includes an oil which may be a skin irritant, it will be less so when part of a selection of essential oils whose *total* is 2 per cent of the final mixture. It may be that the component of the essential oil responsible is present in that one essential oil at, say, 20 per cent, bringing down the percentage of the irritant component in the total mix to an approximate 0.2 per cent! If 5 ml is used on the body each time (e.g. one back massage or five applications to the face), 0.01 ml of the offending component is all that is available for absorption – and remember that only part of that (unlike ingestion) will actually find its way into the body.

CASE EXAMPLE

One of my therapists used five drops each of rosemary and red thyme in 500 ml of water (0.1 per cent) as a rinse on her daughter's hair when she arrived home from school one day with head lice. She applied it slowly and thoroughly, combing the hair intermittently with a fine comb, allowing the hair to dry naturally. When she then combed the hair there were one or two dead lice and some nits. After repeating this procedure, all the nits were killed (there were no more adult parasites).

She gave a mix of the concentrated oils, together with written instructions (always important), to several mothers at the school, who subsequently reported their satisfaction. One mother later told the therapist that her elder son (aged 22) had put some of the concentrated mixture on his pubic hair, which had lice on it (he had not dared tell his mother). He had taken the little bottle, not bothering with the 500 ml of water, but using the oil in its concentrated state. The result was agony for the poor boy – the skin there is particularly sensitive and red thyme is an irritant. He directed the shower head full onto himself, whilst his mother (hearing his cries) fetched some vegetable oil with which to soothe the area and dilute any remaining essential oil (she knew that essential oils did not dissolve properly in water). After a few minutes all was calm – and every louse stone dead!

The severe skin irritation was short lived (approximately 10 minutes) and no permanent harm was done to the boy, but the experience illustrated to that family the power of essential oils and the necessity of using them *as directed*.

Photosensitivity

Phototoxic oils, mainly those of the citrus family (but also including others, e.g. angelica) can cause a reaction on the skin following exposure to sunlight. Furocoumarins (chapter 3) are responsible for photosensitization, making the skin more sensitive to sunlight, hence the sun has an effect more quickly. This is why chemists used to put bergapten – from bergamot oil – into suntanning lotions: this practice has stopped now because it caused uneven tanning in some instances and burning of sensitive skin in others.

Whole bergamot oil is perfectly safe to use so long as the user does not go into strong sunlight (or sunbathe) within the following 2–3 hours.[14]

CASE EXAMPLE

A client of mine arrived one day with a red mark running from her lip to her chin. Asked what had happened, she admitted to using neat bergamot oil on a cold sore at the corner of her mouth just before going on a sunbed. She had used bergamot before, very successfully, for cold sores (two applications usually clearing it), but had never combined ultraviolet exposure with such an application. Bergamot oil is a photosensitizer, thus the melanin cells (responsible for producing the colouring pigment which gives the skin its tanned look), were unusually activated where the bergamot essential oil had run down to her chin.

Her experience taught her a lesson and she now takes care not to expose her skin to the sun or other UV radiation immediately after applying bergamot oil (which she now uses diluted!) After two to three hours, the bergamot oil has penetrated the skin, when it is safe to use a sunbed or go out in the sun.

Allergy and Substance Sensitivity

Our modern times have created an environment which encourages sensitivity and allergy in many people. Years ago, these were not subjects on everybody's lips any more than dieting was (sweets in bulk and rich foods were not abundant in the first half of this century). Nowadays, there is not only a decrease in natural nutrients, but a rapid growth in additives (colourings, food enhancers and preservatives), all of which can be responsible for harmful health reactions. There is also a growth in the number of perfumed items, both household and personal, which may be as hazardous as the food additives, yet are eagerly purchased.

Perfumes have long been a source of allergy or sensitivity reactions – statistics years ago showed that a third of women were sensitive to perfumes. Nowadays, we are surrounded by artificial perfumes in soaps and all toiletries, pot-pourri, women's magazines with perfume samples, household cleaning materials, etc. (even tights and other merchandise are sometimes impregnated with an imperceptible aroma which our receptor cells can pick up and which apparently influences the brand of goods we buy from a store!) As a result, more and more people are finding that they have an 'allergy' to something or other, apart from the fact that synthetic aromas can irritate the nose, aggravate a headache, and affect the breathing of an asthmatic. It is a fact that inhaling car fumes and cigarette smoke (even someone else's) can have a detrimental effect on the health. What many people do not realize (though it has been mentioned in the media) is, that the synthetics used to create the aromas which abound in gift and perfume shops also have a detrimental effect on the body when inhaled. Inhalation takes all substances (harmful or not) right into the body, which, before long, objects and begins to produce symptoms of one sort or another (see below).

Allergies

A lot of confusion abounds nowadays over the use of the word allergy. Everyone blames either an allergic reaction or stress for many of life's problems (the word stress can also be misused).

True allergies are not common and it is now thought that they occur because of a major enzyme deficiency in the digestive system. Normally, the proteins we eat are broken down into amino acids by special enzymes in our digestive systems. When an enzyme required to break down a specific protein is missing, molecules of this unbroken protein enter the blood supply, where they are treated as foreign bodies. This triggers an alarm bell in the immune system, which immediately goes to work to try to expel it. *Only* an unbroken protein can cause this reaction, which usually manifests itself by presenting similar symptoms to those caused by sensitivity or intolerance to certain non-protein substances – hence the confusion.

Known allergens are the proteins in meat, milk, cheese and fish and foods containing any combination of these, like chocolate. Moulds contain proteins, therefore mushrooms too are allergens. Animal hairs, pollen and house dust (which is about 80 per cent composed of human skin cells) are protein based and can cause an allergic reaction. Some washing powders contain proteins and, of particular interest to the reader, wheatgerm oil contains a protein.

CASE EXAMPLE

Several years ago a woman with severe eczema came to see me. She had been on cortisone, on and off, since she was 9 and she was now 26. I was shocked to hear her age, as I had put her down as being about 35–40 (cortisone is very ageing, devouring the body's natural collagen). She was at the end of her tether and had decided, four weeks previously, never to use cortisone again. Naturally, her eczema flared up and resulted in her seeking my advice.

Firstly, we looked at her diet, and removed all cow's milk and dairy products from it (even a little in a cup of tea can sustain an allergy). She agreed to try goat's milk, which is broken down by different enzymes, therefore thoroughly digested. We took out pork (and related foods such as bacon) and all red meats. Fizzy drinks and drinks containing certain 'E number' colorants were forbidden.

Eczema is usually stress based, so we first set out to relieve this by a full aromatherapy treatment at our centre. To help alleviate her symptoms (and improve her skin) I gave her my Special E cream which I felt would help her facial appearance. She also took home some of our silky bath oil containing the same oils. After two weeks we reduced the massage to once a fortnight, then once a month, when she took home our white lotion carrier containing the anti-eczema oils; she used this every night to support the now infrequent massage treatment. The improvement began to show after two or three weeks, during which period her body was getting rid of the cortisone and adjusting to the new diet; I was most delighted with the results on her face and around her eyes, due to using the Special E cream – she had lost ten years and looked a much healthier colour too! She was one of the best clients I ever had regarding diet, sticking closely to the recommended foods; she even wrote to the hotel where she wanted to go on holiday to ask if they would support her diet.

I saw her six months later (because of my travelling, one of my therapists was giving her massage treatment); she had just returned from holiday and was thrilled because she had bought and worn a swimsuit for the first time since she was 12.

Intolerance or Substance Sensitivity

Sensitivity or intolerance can be caused by substances which do not contain proteins, and produces symptoms similar to those resulting from an allergen (these last usually present a stronger reaction).[113] It can sometimes be difficult to discover exactly which substance is causing a particular symptom, as more than one may be involved.

It is believed that sensitivity in people is influenced by the ever-increasing addition of colourings, flavour enhancers, etc. to processed foods and drinks. Coffee, shellfish and strawberries are three well known foods to which people may have an intolerance. Washing powders and perfumes are also notorious culprits.

Essential oils, particularly when adulterated in some way with chemicals, can produce a reaction on some people known to be sensitive to perfumes. It is in such a person's interest to carry out a test as follows with the oils to be used. Up to four oils can be tested at once, but do not forget to make a note of which oil is where on your skin!

Simply place one drop on a small area of your upper chest or in the crook of your arm and leave it for 12 hours. If there is no irritation or redness, the probability is that you are not sensitive to the oil.

The symptoms of allergy/sensitivity are widespread and can be missed or misunderstood by practitioners, who then take a symptomatic approach, which may fail altogether or simply relieve the symptoms temporarily.

Possible symptoms may be

mental – such as depression, confusion or exhaustion and/or
physical – like asthma, constipation, diarrhoea, dizziness, hay fever, headaches, palpitations, rhinitis, stomach ulcers, swelling, skin irritations such as eczema or dermatitis . . . a long list!

Sensitization

Some substances, like hair colourings, have the ability suddenly to cause an intolerance; a reaction may occur after several years of eating or using a particular item (such as hair colouring; which is why conscientious hairdressers usually test their clients from time to time before administering a colour).

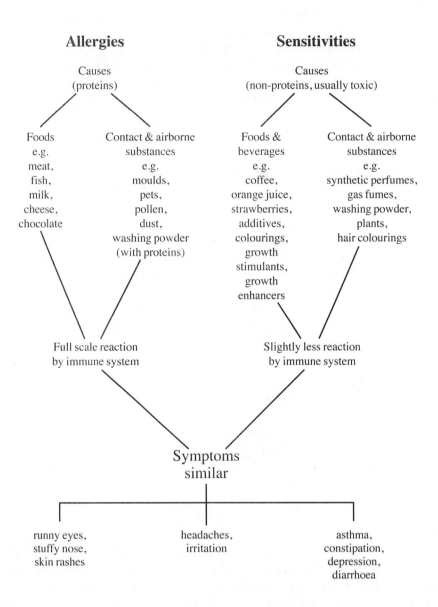

FIGURE 6.1: Symptoms caused by allergies and sensitivities

Several essential oils may be skin sensitizers, especially when insufficiently diluted. Research results can be misleading, if the diluted isolated chemical is used for tests on skin sensitization, rather than the whole, diluted essential oil (as in aromatherapy). Aromatherapists should therefore place more emphasis on research papers where the *whole* oil has been used, rather than tests using isolated fractions of the oil. It is possible for an aromatherapist suddenly to develop sensitivity to an essential oil – I have only heard of this twice and in both cases lavender was the offending oil, possibly because it is used in nearly every treatment by some therapists. I also know of one case where the reaction was purely psychosomatic and when tested unknown to herself with the same oil, from the same bottle, there was no reaction whatsoever (a perfect illustration of the power of the mind, which had told her she was allergic to lavender because of past experience with lavender-fragranced products).

We have already learned that tests carried out on animals have presented results which do not match those done on humans – because our skin is of a different nature, there is no reaction.[9]

The International Fragrance Association (IFRA), because of the nature of the products they formulate, have carried out many tests on skin reactions, using both whole essential oils and the offending isolate (see reference to cinnamon earlier in the chapter). As a result (and with the advice of a perfumer friend of mine) I was able to add, to a recipe containing lemongrass (whose aldehyde content can cause sensitization), a measured amount of an oil containing a high percentage of dextro-limonene, to cancel the effect of the citral (see page 125). Synergy again? This is why it is often safe to use an oil or lotion on the skin if it is formulated by someone with experience, even if it may contain a potentially hazardous oil.

It is not possible to list all essential oils which may be sensitizers – somewhere, someone may find they have a susceptibility to a seemingly innocent oil; the main ones tested are in Table 4 (page 126). The Latin name of the oil concerned should be noted, together with the variety or chemotype which contains the constituent chemical(s) responsible for any hazard, as some varieties or chemotypes of the same species, or from a different part of the plant, may be innocent.

I would like to close this chapter by citing one or two instances where insufficient knowledge has resulted in the incorrect application of essential oils in hospitals. These have been provided by a conscientious and caring aromatherapist/nurse, who is employed by the National Health Service to supervise aromatherapy treatments in several hospitals.

CASE EXAMPLE 1

(This case shows clearly the negligent way in which some essential oils are marketed.)

A qualified nurse working on a post-surgical ward was found to be using neat essential oil of nutmeg on a client's foot. In an interview she explained that in the leaflet accompanying some oils she had bought it stated that 'nutmeg is a warming oil'.

The oils were purchased through a shopping catalogue and were of poor quality. This nurse had no qualification in aromatherapy, had not referred to a book on the subject, and had been applying several drops of the oil, undiluted, once a day for six days.

The episode was discovered before the oil was used long enough to cause any harmful effects.

Author's comment: Nutmeg, with its content of myristicin (a phenolic ether), is a powerful brain relaxant and should not be on sale 'over the counter'. This same 100 per cent nutmeg oil may have been bought (and used incorrectly) by several other members of the general public – the label simply said 'Nutmeg Oil' so it was not easy to identify.

CASE EXAMPLE 2

A nursing assistant had been given a bottle of Roman chamomile by a friend, who told her that the oil was good for eye infections.

A patient on a day unit had 'pink eye' – conjunctivitis – and this nursing assistant put two drops in his eye.

The patient was taken to casualty and the oil washed out.

This sad episode ended by no further aromatherapy treatments being allowed on that particular ward.

Author's comment: It is not known whether or not the friend gave verbal instructions regarding the necessity of diluting the essential oil – particularly for use in the eyes; *written* instructions are necessary when giving advice and it seems that neither the friend nor the nursing assistant had sought qualified advice or thoroughly read a book on aromatherapy.

This apart, the eye area is particularly delicate and it is advised that it is not bathed or treated with self-blended essential oils. (I have myself formulated an extremely safe product for soothing dry, irritated or tired eyes.)

I was at a dinner when an 'aromatherapist' put a drop of Roman chamomile into the eye of one of the guests. Until I asked what was the matter, the 'victim', suffering intensely, was being told by the 'therapist' that the stinging should 'soon go off'! The best antidote for neat essential oil in the eye is vegetable carrier oil, as this immediately dilutes the essential oil. The eye should then be rinsed thoroughly with water for several minutes (which was the only thing we could do for the girl at the dinner; after five or six minutes of continuous rinsing, her eye was almost back to normal).

I would like to assure people that no permanent damage is done if essential oil accidentally gets into the eye, so long as it is rinsed out immediately (preferably adding vegetable oil first) – it is the intense stinging which is so upsetting.

CASE EXAMPLE 3

A nursing assistant using the essential oil of peppermint in a bath, was told that this would be cooling (which it is, under normal use), but he thought two to three drops to be nothing in such a large amount of water – so administered more than 20.

The patient had a somewhat unpleasant tingling on the legs and a burning sensation in the genital area.

This client, although soon back to normal, will not now have anything to do with aromatherapy treatments.

Author's comment: At the risk of repeating an earlier part of this chapter, I must emphasize that much of the misunderstanding of the strength of neat essential oils stems from the fact that *diluted* oils were introduced into the market (well before undiluted essential oils) in 8–10 ml bottles *with a drop dispenser*, and without giving a content list or percentage dilution. To sell such a small amount of diluted oil is in any case ridiculous – one bath or back massage and it is half, or all, gone! Had the nursing assistant above used a bottle of diluted peppermint, 20 drops would barely have been enough!

When neat essential oils, in the same bottle and drop dispenser, made their appearance (much better value for money!) who was to know they were so different (same bottle, same dropper)? The amount to be used was thrown into complete confusion, exacerbated by the fact that both diluted oils (particularly) and neat oils were sold with insufficient information on the label. Pricewise, the former contains around 97 per cent of vegetable oil (much lower priced) and yet may be sold at the same price as 100 per cent essential oil (depending on the oil concerned).

CASE EXAMPLE 4

A nurse came to me and asked about carrier oils. She said that she had been using a vegetable oil, but that within a short while of applying it to the client, it became sticky. I asked to see the oil used, and it turned out to be 'Crisp and Dry'!

She said, 'This experience has made me see the necessity of having correct and precise product information.'

Author's comment: I could not agree more! (see Carrier Oils – chapter 8).

7 Essential Oils: Storage, Carriers and Methods of Use

Storage

Everyone is used to seeing essential oils in coloured, rather than clear, bottles, and there is a good reason for this. Essential oils deteriorate in sunlight – faster at the blue end of the spectrum than the red. This is why amber brown bottles are considered to be the best, even though I think blue ones are more attractive. (Black would probably be even better!)

If your oils are in a blue bottle it is necessary to keep them in the dark; brown ones too are best kept in the dark, though it is not quite as important, so long as they are not in direct sunlight; windowsills, sunny shelves (and shelves on radiators) etc., should be avoided. A warm place is not good for essential oils, especially if the bottle is not full; the oxygen in the air gap can attack the oil and cause deterioration.

As essential oils are volatile, replace the cap after use: otherwise, not only will the oil gradually evaporate, but the lighter molecules will disappear first, thus slightly altering the composition of the oil.

How long will essential oils keep? There are many differing views on this, but in perfect storage conditions – i.e. in brown bottles in a cool place and without an air space – about six years. There are instances of essential oil keeping quite well for 30–40 years. As none of us needs to keep them as long as that, the average keeping time should be two to three years – long enough not to worry about a 'best before' date, so long as the bottling date is known.

Citrus peel oils do not have such a long life, because the aldehydes tend to turn into acids. This can be delayed by keeping them in the fridge, but then the waxes (not present in distilled oils) may be precipitated. This does not affect the therapeutic chemicals – it just makes the oil opaque.

The waxes can be filtered out – warming will not make them go back into solution.

Absolutes and resins have a shorter life than essential oils, because they tend to thicken slightly with age and the smell of the solvents used becomes more apparent.

When essential oils are mixed into oil or lotion carriers, the shelf life of that product is only as long as that of the carrier. In a vegetable carrier oil, the keeping qualities are considerably reduced to nine or perhaps 12 months at most. As with absolutes, the smell changes, this time when the vegetable oil has gone rancid (the effects of the essential oil, as far as is known, are not impaired by this). When the oil is added to a 'long-life' lotion, its keeping qualities are the same as that of the pure essential oil on its own.

Storage rules regarding light, heat and airtight closure apply even more to essential oils in carrier oil.

Caution   Never leave a bottle of pure essential oil on a polished or painted surface or certain types of plastic; these may be susceptible to the chemicals in the oil and if so, would be damaged.

Carriers

Carriers are anything which 'carry' essential oils into the body, and are not restricted to vegetable oils and lotions. Air is a carrier – when you inhale an essential oil from a tissue it is not the concentrated essence alone which travels up the nose – it is accompanied by molecules of air from the atmosphere. Water is a carrier, and when essential oils are put into warm water, the effects are twofold, because the heat releases the aromatic molecules more quickly. All the aromatherapy skin creams and lotions, shampoos and bath products available now are simply carriers to enable the essential oils contained in them to be absorbed into the human system.

Penetration

How do essential oils penetrate the human system?

Through the Nose   Inhalation is the quickest method by which essential oils enter the body and take effect. The surrounding warm, moist air carries the tiny molecules up the nose as we breathe in. This wonderful piece of 'apparatus' is the only organ with direct access to the brain (which is responsible for influencing our feelings and actions) thus making the effect of aromas by inhalation exceptionally important.

There are minute 'hairs' called cilia right at the top of the nose, from which special signals commence their journey to the brain. The air we breathe in passes over these cilia, which are equipped with millions of special individually shaped indentations, each one accepting a specific aroma molecule, which fits into it rather like a key in a lock.[114] When the aroma 'key' is locked in its own space, a signal is transmitted from receptor cells to the olfactory bulb and hence to the limbic and hypothalamus (sections of the brain designed to process this information).

Neurochemicals are then released which are passed on, via the nervous system, to relax or stimulate it – according to the aroma. They also affect the body physically, which is why essential oils are so effective for the relief of pain, such as that experienced with headaches, arthritis, indigestion, etc. To illustrate – if you have not eaten for a while and you smell food cooking, instructions are sent to your digestive system to prepare itself – and you feel hungry! Not everyone possesses every possible shape of indentation in their cilia, which explains why some people are unable to smell certain aromas.

Very little of the oil released into the air to be inhaled goes up the nose (most floats into the room) and probably only a small proportion of this reaches the brain or lungs, and from there, the rest of the body. I mention this in order to show how little essential oil actually goes into the body and, therefore, how little is needed to have an effect.

Ingestion   The essential oils, in a suitable carrier, travel through the body from the stomach – their first port of call. Used this way, all the essential oil is immediately absorbed into the body; this is one reason why it is recommended not to take essential oils internally without the advice of a well-qualified aromatherapist working with a doctor or an aromatologist.

Through the Skin   Essential oil molecules are extremely minute and are therefore able to penetrate the skin via the hair follicles and sweat glands.[115] It is thought that they can also permeate between the skin cells, through the lipids (saturated fats) and, as essential oils are soluble in fat, they can enter the dermis this way. Once there, they can reach the tiny blood capillaries and lymph, from where they are transported around the body by the circulatory system. Urine tested an hour after applying essential oil on the back of the hand has been found to contain the oil applied. There have been many tests which corroborate this finding, including checking exhaled air.

Applied to the skin, it is thought that even less of the total oil used is absorbed into the body; the hands rubbing in the oil and the skin receiving it are both warm, causing many of the volatile molecules to evaporate before they can find their way through the skin surfaces. As use on the skin is one of the major routes into the body that aromatherapy employs in the UK (and countries to which it has spread since), the hazards and toxicity questions raised against essential oils resulting from tests using excessive doses internally hardly seem to apply – it is those hazards (which are fortunately few) presented by use on the skin with which we must concern ourselves (see chapter 6) especially if fractionated or adulterated oils are used!

Air as a Carrier

Inhalation of essential oils works mainly on the mind, encouraging the body to heal itself. Thus, when depression, stress, jealousy or over-tiredness are causing physical imbalances in the body, the relaxing or stimulating effects of essential oils can start us on the road to good health. Some typical examples of health problems which can be helped by inhalation are headaches, insomnia, breathing difficulties of every kind, nausea and hormonal problems.

As well as influencing the brain when inhaled, the oils have direct access to the mucous membrane of the nose and to the lungs, hence it is possible to obtain relief from catarrh, sinusitis, bronchitis and psychosomatic illnesses like asthma.

From your Hands
In an emergency, a speedy method is to put one drop of essential oil into your palm, rub your hands together briefly (which warms the oil), cup them over the nose, keeping them away from the eyes, and take a deep breath.

From a Tissue
One of the most effective ways to inhale essential oils, particularly if an immediate reaction is required, is to place a few drops on a paper tissue (kitchen tissues are best) or a handkerchief and take three **deep** breaths.

The tissue can then be placed inside the shirt or blouse, so that molecules of essential oil, evaporating due to the body warmth, can continue gently to be inhaled.

From Pot-Pourri

If you have flowers or attractive leaves in your garden, put some fresh, small petals and/or leaves into a screw-top jam jar and sprinkle them with the pure essential oils of your choice. Shake well, then place them in a decorative bowl or on a pretty plate. Although not as long-lasting as artificially perfumed pot-pourri, the aroma is fresher and better for your health.

From a Basin of Hot Water

For colds and coughs put two or three drops of essential oil into hot (not boiling) water and breathe in slowly – the heat makes the oils evaporate quickly, increasing the strength of the aroma. It is important not to use more drops as the strength could make you cough – keep your eyes closed to protect them from the powerful vapours.

Caution   If you are asthmatic this may 'catch your breath' (unless you try one drop). You could try inhaling from your hands instead (see above).

From a Spray

A good way of inhaling essential oils (with water as an additional carrier) is to spray a room using a plant spray bottle. Put about half a pint of water into the bottle, add 10 or 12 drops of essential oil and shake well before spraying the room.

From a Vaporizer

In Europe, great emphasis has been placed for years on the vaporizer, which is now very popular in Britain too. It is a lovely way to benefit from the effects of essential oils – in fact, the whole room (sometimes the whole house) smells wonderful and everyone can enjoy the aroma. Many people use them every day, to keep infections at bay over the winter months, to relax the brain or body after a stressful day, or even to relax or stimulate your guests at a party to set the mood! They can also be used as a stimulant before sex if you have difficulties in that direction – a multitude of stress-related problems can be gently helped this way without feeling you are making a special effort.

The safest vaporizer is an electric one, especially where children and old people are concerned. These are more expensive, and provided you take care to position them well, vaporizers using a night-light or candle are adequate, a multitude of different sizes and designs being available. Keep the little 'cup' topped up with water, replacing the essential oils as and when necessary otherwise the heavier molecules of the oil will be left till the end without water, and these can have an acrid smell as they burn off. The number of drops to be used is not crucial – it depends on the size of the room and how long you want the aroma to continue.

If you do not possess a vaporizer you can put the essential oils into a bowl of very hot water, though this method is not so efficient (the water soon becomes cold). To lengthen the effect, you can put them on a saucer over the bowl, when the water can easily be replaced. This method works best if put on a sunny table, windowsill or warm radiator.

During wintertime, make use of the radiator. Put the essential oil onto a crumpled tissue or a cotton wall ball and place this anywhere in firm contact with the heat.

Caution   Essential oils are very volatile and can burst into flames if near a flame, or strong source of heat. Hollow rings are available for vaporizing essential oils over a light bulb – these are potentially dangerous in my opinion. Extreme care needs to be taken with them, and oil should never be added while the ring is in position; if any oil drips onto the bulb itself, or the fitting, it could burst into flames. Similarly, adding essential oil to the hot wax of an already lit candle (although in theory an effective method) could be hazardous, perhaps resulting in the loss of eyebrows, so beware!

People using vaporizers for non-therapeutic reasons often use perfume quality oils, or even synthetics, purely to benefit from the aroma. Artificial molecules also have an effect on your system. I, personally, am so used to the clear aromas of pure oils that I find some perfume oils cloying, and can no longer enjoy being in a shop where synthetic fragrances abound in soap, bath bubbles and pot-pourri. One day, I intend to add true essential oils to a non-caustic pure soap I have found in France – and I already dry petals for pot-pourri.

Water as a Carrier

Baths

The most popular method of using essential oils with water is in the bath. Six to eight drops will give a beneficial effect and, if using oils already diluted in a carrier (as in most commercial products), one or two teaspoonfuls will be necessary depending on the percentage of essential oils (if it tells you!)

Essential oils diluted in carrier oils for the bath are useful if you have a dry skin though they tend to leave a greasy mark around the bath (better to treat yourself to cream or use a body lotion with essential oils for dry skin afterwards). For health problems, a *macerated* oil of benefit to that problem, together with essential oils, is worth the inevitable oily ring (see chapter 8 – calendula, carrot, hypericum, lime blossom, melissa and mullein).

Essential oils can be dissolved first in cream, yoghurt, the top of the milk (a better solvent than fat-free milk) or honey. Cleopatra used sour asses' milk, but you may have difficulty procuring that! Claudine Luu, an essential oil expert with whom I teach aromatherapy in France, finds powdered milk to be one of the best media; put the essential oils into the milk powder with just sufficient water to make a paste, then into the bath.

For all methods it is important to run the bath first (to the temperature required) before adding the essential oils, swishing the water thoroughly to disperse them. You can then climb in, relax and let the oils do their work. Stay in for at least ten minutes to inhale those molecules evaporating from the surface, and for those in the water to penetrate your skin.

As absolute and resinoid oils always have a little of the solvent left in them (the amount depends on the quality of the oil – see chapter 2), they are best not used in the bath unless blended with other essential oils first (or a teaspoonful of vegetable oil, honey or cream). Added on their own, they tend to sink to the bottom and, because of their concentrated nature, the fabric of the bath may be affected (depending on the type of plastic from which it is made).

Foot and Hand Baths

If your hands or feet need help, whether for swelling, pain, heat, athlete's foot, or whatever, ten minutes in a foot or handbath containing six to eight drops of the appropriate essential oils will soon bring relief. It is a good idea to have a kettle of hot water beside you to add to the bowl, for when the water begins to get cold. For added luxury, you can apply a lotion containing the same oils to your feet and lower legs afterwards. Footbaths can also be used to help relieve headaches or other minor ailments, because of the effect of the oils on the foot reflexes.

Sitz Baths

A sitz bath with essential oils is a simple way of dealing with haemor-rhoids, thrush, stitches after childbirth, etc. (as an alternative to a conventional bath). Tea tree is the miracle oil for thrush, as it not only is extremely effective, but is also non-aggressive on both the skin and mucous membranes. Put three to four drops into a bowl of warm water and sit in it for ten minutes. For stitches, use two drops of cypress and two drops lavender; for haemorrhoids substitute one drop of peppermint for the two of lavender.

Jacuzzis and Hydrotherapy Baths

Many people own jacuzzi or hydrotherapy baths and their advantage over a normal bath is that, because of the movement of the water, the essential oil molecules are circulated continually and dispersed evenly throughout the whole bath. This gives them access to the skin of the whole body, not just that in contact with the surface of the water, which means that oil molecules are being absorbed into the entire submerged skin surface. In addition, the evaporating molecules are being inhaled from the surface of the water as in a normal bath.

Essential oils diluted in a vegetable oil should not be used in a hydrotherapy bath, because, as the water is continually passing through the pump, the vegetable oil will gradually coat the pipes, which are not easy to clean! Neat essential oils do not have this effect and can be used with safety. They should not be added until the bath is filled and the pump switched on; this ensures immediate dispersion of the oils.

The number of drops of essential oil required in a hydrotherapy bath varies slightly with the size of the bath. A bath designed for only one person will require from six to eight drops, whereas nine or 10 drops could be added to one which can accommodate two or three people.

Saunas

Essential oils can be put into the water which is tossed onto the stones. It is wonderful with any oil, and with pine (an air disinfectant), eucalyptus and a little peppermint it is most effective for a blocked nose! Because the air in a sauna is hot (80-100°C), two or three drops of essential oil are sufficient.

It is not advisable to have a sauna just before an aromatherapy massage, as the exhaling pores of your skin will have difficulty in accepting the incoming molecules of essential oil, so little benefit will be derived from them.

Showers
People write about using essential oils in the shower, but it is not an easy thing to do! Some say to put the essential oils onto a sponge or face cloth while in the shower, others to apply the oils in a carrier all over the body before stepping into the shower. A shower gel or shampoo containing essential oils may be a better way, though whichever way is used, the oils are washed off almost immediately. There may be some benefit from inhaling them briefly before they disappear down the plug hole, but for full benefit I much prefer my bath!

Compresses
These can be used successfully for a number of problems, insect bites, arthritic joints, period or stomach pains, headaches, sprains, varicose veins, etc. Decide first whether you need a hot or a cold compress; where there is inflammation and heat, a cold one is best (ice cubes can be added to cold water); for a dull ache, use a warm one.

The cloth used should be a natural fibre, such as cotton (handkerchiefs or old tea towels are ideal). The amount of water used is important and should be chosen according to the size of the area to be treated (for a finger compress an egg cupful is sufficient). Add your essential oils and use just enough water to soak into the compress (from two drops for a septic finger up to eight drops for an abdominal pain). Stir well to disperse the essential oils.

Lower the centre of the cotton into the basin slowly to absorb any floating oil, then lightly squeeze out any surplus water and lay it onto the problem area, holding in place with a strip of cling film (if practical). With a cool compress, a sealed plastic bag of crushed ice cubes (or pack of frozen peas) placed on top and held in place would be helpful (it will need periodic changing); with a warm one, wrap a strip of material such as wool, a thermal garment, or even tights, over the cling film. To keep a compress in place on an arm or leg, a sock or a leg from old tights is ideal.

Leave the compress in place for at least an hour, or overnight for something septic.

Gargles and Mouthwashes

Essential oils are very effective for voice loss – I use them if my voice becomes croaky when lecturing to large audiences for three or four successive days. I gargle in front of everyone (with my back to the audience!) so that they can hear the immediate effect. For sore throats, and colds which may go onto the chest, a twice daily gargle is extremely helpful.

Put two to three drops of essential oil into a glass and half fill with water (I use soothing oils like sandalwood with Roman chamomile, geranium or cypress). Stir well, take a mouthful, gargle and spit it out. Stir again and repeat. It is important to stir before each mouthful to re-disperse the oils.

The procedure for mouthwashes is exactly the same, except that the liquid is swished around inside your mouth for a few seconds instead of at the back of your throat. For enhanced effect, roll it around for a full minute before spitting out.

Beverages (Water and Tea)

Many people do not like drinking water on its own – even the bottled variety. When we go to Mediterranean countries like Egypt, we put two drops of fennel into each litre bottle of spring water to keep our stomachs happy! We shake it well each time before drinking, and even clean our teeth with it. It tastes rather like weak Pernod!

If you are trying to slim, use two to three drops of grapefruit oil to a litre of water and drink 2–3 glasses per day between meals; one or two of my clients have found this helpful (together with careful eating), especially those who cannot remember to apply an essential oil mix in a lotion or carrier oil regularly to their body twice a day.

When I first entered the world of aromatherapy I used to recommend essential oil teas to all my clients, giving them one after they had had their massage treatment. When essential oils are to be ingested it is vital that the distilled or expressed oils used are of therapeutic quality (resins and absolutes should never be used). With the plethora of sometimes dubious essential oils on the general market it is difficult to recommend teas as a method of use. Also, the code of ethics of the aromatherapy associations does not allow therapists to prescribe oils for clients' internal use as medicines (though they can and do take them themselves), as their insurance does not cover this aspect. Apart from this, it would be difficult to control the number of drops a client used, or the number of weeks of self-treatment. However, tea is not a medicine, and is expected to have a pleasant taste; if it did not, it would be thrown away.

If you drink Earl Grey tea, you ingest a minute amount of bergamot oil in each cup and you can make your own, using tannin-free china tea. To make it (and other flavours), put two or three drops of essential oil onto the teabag (or in a tea-egg with the tea leaves), pour on approximately one litre of water, stir well and remove the tea. The tea tastes best (and is better for the health) without the addition of milk.

Do not put a drop of essential oil directly into a cup of tea – the taste will be too strong, and the oil will not be dispersed effectively.

If you decide to use this method, I must emphasize the use of therapeutic quality oils only, and no absolutes or resins. A few small essential oil bottles certainly take up a lot less room than many different flavours of tea and in the long run are less expensive!

For indigestion and other digestive disorders, like constipation and diarrhoea, a cup of tea two or three times a day is more pleasant than tablets. Urinary tract problems, like cystitis and urethritis, react favourably too. I know many people who have found teas to be helpful for the above and also for insomnia and arthritic pain.

Herbal teas (or tisanes as they are sometimes called) are becoming more popular every day – some supermarkets even stock a few. A French colleague of mine makes herbal teas for specific health conditions, like diabetes, overweight, high blood pressure, arthritis, etc. She has just obtained a licence for these, which means she can now distribute them. These herbal teas present a much better method for ingesting a plant's benefits than using aromatherapy internally as a medicine – up to ten different types of plant are carefully chosen and mixed for each one, ensuring an effective balance.

Vegetable Oils and Bland Lotion as Carriers

Vegetable Oils
Except in an emergency, such as a burn, the prevention of a bruise after a knock, a wasp sting, a deep cut or a burst spot, essential oils should not be

used in their neat state on the skin; they should always be mixed into a carrier of some sort.

The most well-known carriers for this purpose are fixed vegetable oils into which essential oils readily dissolve. Many different ones are on the market today, each having its own special benefit to the skin (see chapter 8). Mineral oil (e.g. baby oil) is not a good carrier; it is protective to the skin and ideal for babies in that it keeps moisture out, which makes it difficult for the essential oils to get in!

Though used for self-application (i.e. to the skin), and sometimes in the bath (see 'baths' above) the primary purpose of a vegetable carrier oil is for massage, which requires a medium allowing for continuous and prolonged movement by the hands on the body, without dragging and without slipping. If the consistency of the oil is correct and an accurate amount of oil is applied, there will be no drag or slip.

N.B. When using a diluted oil from a bottle for self-application, may I suggest that you place your fingers over the top of the bottle, tipping it up against them. Apply to the area requiring help, then repeat should you need more oil. This way, you will not take more than is necessary.

A single body massage takes between 10 and 20 ml of oil, depending on the size (and hairiness) of the person being massaged (quantities are given below). It is always better to mix less rather than more, as any left over will contain the essential oil which was part of the treatment. If there is not enough oil to complete the massage, a little extra plain carrier oil can be always be used.

Lotion

It is easier, when using essential oils on yourself, to put them into a non-greasy, non-staining, vegetable based lotion rather than a vegetable oil. If you need the treatment on your hands, a bottle containing an oil mixture can slip from your fingers as you pick it up to replace the cap; this does not happen with a lotion. Also, it is easy to take too much oil and, if you need to apply your mixture every day, your clothes may eventually become discoloured by the excess. Finally, and this is why I prefer using my carrier lotion on myself, a lotion disappears into the skin after a few seconds of rubbing, leaving it soft and smooth, without any greasy feeling.

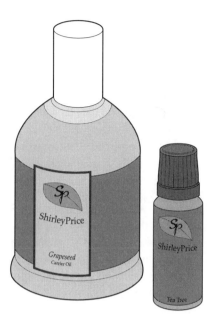

FIGURE 7.1:

Adding Essential Oils to Carrier Oils and Lotion

If you know you are going to be using the same massage oil or lotion every week (or every day if you are using it for self-application), it is better to pre-mix this into a 50 or 100 ml bottle. The recipe below is for 100 ml, which is easier to divide into smaller quantities. You may need to refer to chapter 8 for the properties, stability and viscosity of any vegetable oil or oils you want to use as the base.

Mixing into a Vegetable Oil in Quantity   Take a 100 ml brown glass bottle (available from your chemist) and put into it 30–40 drops of the essential oils you have chosen. Wheatgerm oil (a natural preservative) should then be added to increase the keeping qualities, the amount depending on the base oil (or oils), and should never be less than 5 per cent (5 ml in 100 ml); 10 per cent is better and up to 20 per cent (20ml in 100 ml) can be added if desired. Then add any special vegetable oil or oils you feel you need, almost up to the top of the bottle (manufacturers always leave 10 per cent extra space) and not using more than 20 per cent of another heavy oil, such as avocado. Screw the top on firmly, shake once or twice, and label it with the recipe, the condition it is formulated to help and the date. It is then easier to adjust (or retain) the recipe next time round, and the date will help you to know if you made too much or too little.

Mixing into a Lotion Base in Quantity   Use the same recipe as for a mix using an oil base. Any special carrier oils you may need must be added to the lotion first, a little at a time, and mixed well. Fill your bottle with only three-quarters of the required amount of lotion (or lotion and special carrier oil) add the essential oils and shake well. Add the rest of the lotion, leaving a 10 per cent air gap so that a final good shake can be given to ensure an even blend of oils and lotion.

Mixing for One Treatment or Self-Applied Massage   A good guide as to how much carrier oil to use for one complete body massage is as follows: for women, use their (British) dress size, e.g. for size 10 use 10 ml, 12 use 12 ml, and so on; for men (with average hairiness), use half their chest size, e.g. for size 40 use 20 ml, 44 use 22 ml, and so on (these quantities are for someone with a normal skin). For a back massage only, you will need about a third of these amounts, but you may still add the same number of drops of essential oil, as they will be shared around the whole body through the circulatory system.

Take a slightly smaller amount of the lotion, vegetable oil or oils of your choice than you think you will need (wheatgerm will not be needed for its stabilizing powers), then add your essential oils – four to six drops in 10 ml; six to eight drops in 20 ml.

The number of drops of essential oil used should vary in direct proportion to the body weight and must also take into consideration the age as well as the mental and physical states of the person. Following these principles, and as a general guide, children will therefore need only half as many drops as an adult: the very old should be given the same number of drops as children; babies should have only half the number of drops used on children.

The number of drops recommended is never exact (there is no recognized precise figure – typically given, as for example, 6–8 or 15–20, etc.) and it may be better that anyone with severe mental difficulties should be given the lower figure.

Mixing Pure Essential Oils   Once you have found a blend of essential oils you want to use on a regular basis (and/or which is beneficial to your health), it is much simpler to mix them together in a small bottle with a dropper. For instance, should you find that two drops of sandalwood and four each of geranium and lavender are the best oils for you, you would simply put a zero at the end of your number (making it 20 and 40 drops), or change the drops into ml (2 and 4 ml) if you have a measure. From this blend (or mix) you can easily dispense and use whatever number of drops you need.

Cream

I would suggest that you can add essential oils to any cream, but as I would not know whether the contents would be compatible with essential oils, this is difficult. I produce a moisture cream without essential oils for those who wish to add their own to help particular problems. It is much easier to allay the symptoms of something like chronic sinus problems, broken veins or persistent headaches at the same time as you moisturize your face and neck, rather than having to apply something else as well (or even forgetting to do it regularly!) I once broke my nose while teaching at a health farm (I fell over some chairs in the dark, and did not realize at the time that I had broken it). The bone reset itself slightly incorrectly and I developed catarrh. I decided to try anticatarrhal essential oils in my moisture cream base to make sure of treating the catarrh daily – and it works wonderfully well.

Hints on the Regular Use of Essential Oils

Essential oils are synergistic (from the Greek, *syn* = together and *ergon* = work). Each essential oil is a synergistic mix in itself, the chemical components all working together to give the end effects, which is another reason for using only whole, un-tampered with essential oils.[116] It is also a proven fact that the effects of two or three oils together is greater than the sum of their individual effects.[117] I have always advocated using more than one essential oil (often three or four), which also provides a chance to create a pleasing blend of aromas.

A question I am often asked at lectures and by students is how many drops of essential oil can one use each day. If you are using them externally, every day, a total of six drops of a mix of oils would be well within the safety limits (not six drops of *one* oil – this would depend on the oil chosen). It is possible to receive approximately 0.1 of a drop each day from your moisturizer and the same for other skin care items; one or two from your bath (remember, only part of the oil is directed into your body); 0.01 from a room vaporizer; 0.5 from self-application for a health problem – leaving at least three drops still not used – perhaps a massage once a week will cover that! I am setting it out like this to show you that it is difficult to use too many drops every day. Remember that, unlike ingestion, only a small percentage of the drops find their way into your system, so your body is probably accepting less than I have implied (see 'Penetration' at the beginning of this chapter). In fact, using essential oils every day keeps you healthy (the staff who work in our laboratory, and who are inhaling essential oils all day, are rarely off work). If, on the other hand, apart from your skin care items, you only use essential oils intermittently, e.g. when you have a cold, insect bite, period pain, a massage once a month, etc., it is safe to use up to 12 drops, made up from several oils, in any one day (for the limited time you will need them), having first made absolutely sure that none of the oils you have chosen are contra-indicated for your particular condition or state of health.

A question which interests aromatherapists is whether it is good for them to use essential oils all day in massage. The amount inhaled during a treatment is very small and the palms of the hands will be excreting more than they can take in, due to the the warmth (the massage hopefully gives the client most of the four to six drops used). Even if the therapist were lucky enough to 'steal' a little of this from each client, it could not add up to be excessive in any one day!

I cannot say this often enough: careful and normal moderate use of essential oils (as with most things in life) brings only benefit.

8 *Carrier Oils*

Vegetable oils are probably the most familiar carriers used in aromatherapy and deserve to be gone into in detail, as they have interesting properties of their own. Unlike essential oils, vegetable oils are greasy and come under the heading of 'fixed' oils, which do not evaporate; they leave an oily mark on absorbent paper.

Carrier oils can be divided into three main groups – 'basic' oils (the highest proportion of a massage mix) – 'specialized' fixed oils (more often used as a percentage of the main mix – perhaps too thick or costly to use on their own) and macerated oils (plant extracts in a basic fixed oil).

Basic carrier oils are much paler in colour than specialized oils such as avocado (dark green) and wheatgerm oil (rich golden brown). Jojoba is an exception – it is pale, but is a liquid *wax*, not a triglyceride oil, and is in the more expensive class of carriers.

Vegetable oils can be extracted from nuts or seeds by two methods. One is cold pressing, which is costly and executed on a comparatively small scale. Hot extraction (the second method) is a much larger industry, a more complicated process, yet paradoxically, less expensive, as the demand is so great and a considerably higher yield of oil is produced (albeit not such good quality). The two industries are usually separate, a cold-pressing factory not carrying out hot extraction as well.

Carrier oils for aromatherapy should be cold pressed, though this is a slight misnomer, as a certain amount of heat is employed to help release the oil, usually not higher than 60°C. The nuts or seeds are placed in a horizontal press with an enormous 'screw'. As this turns, the oil is squeezed out and drips into a trough below – a fascinating process to watch. The first oil to be collected is known as 'virgin pressed' (olive oil is commercially available in virgin and second pressings). Natural heat is generated as the pressure increases to force out more oil, but careful watch is kept to see that it does not reach 70–80°C (60 degrees is the limit allowed in France – no limit in the UK). If higher than this, the oil cannot be classed as cold pressed. After pressing, the oil is filtered in successive cotton cloths and finally through a paper filter.

The remaining 'cake' is sold to the farming industry to put into animal feed, or to factories carrying out hot extraction for the food industry. When these factories buy original seeds or nuts, the first extraction is carried out at high temperatures – up to 200°C. The remaining cake, together with that from the oil pressing factories, is mixed with a solvent such as petrol, to extract any residual oil. During the complicated refining process which follows, involving an even greater heat, the colour is bleached out, natural odour and all flavour being also removed. Refining can have a destructive effect on the aroma, vitamin and enzyme content of the oil. Colour is added at the end of the process to give a standardized shade and firms who wish to advertise vitamin content add these too.

Vegetable oils extracted this way are labelled as 'pure', which seems highly suspect – but quite legal! Nevertheless, refining does give an oil more stability and greater keeping qualities; of great importance to the food industry, but at what a cost!

The above explanation should partly explain why cold pressed and unrefined oils, although more desirable for therapeutic use, are more expensive than heat extracted and refined oils. As the vast majority of buyers require refined oils, the huge quantities they order also brings the price of refined oils down to a very low level.

General Points About Carrier Oils

All cold pressed carrier oils have specific beneficial effects on bodily health, as they contain vitamins, minerals and therapeutic fatty acids in varying degrees, and recently many aromatherapists have shown a greater interest in these health benefits. When taken internally, all the health benefits can be felt (with regular use), including the improvement of dry skin, eczema etc., which are often symptoms of an inner cause.

Many believe, incorrectly, that if an ingested vegetable oil is beneficial to certain systems of the body, it follows that all these benefits will be passed on through massage. Vegetable oils are comprised of much larger molecules than essential oils, and on the whole are unable to pass through the skin. Even though we may be able to absorb the vitamins and minerals etc. through application[118] the benefits to the skin itself are quite numerous.

The properties of vegetable oils relating to the skin can be of vital importance, especially as they comprise at least 95 per cent of any massage mix, and should always be taken into account when treating skin conditions – it is no use using a carrier whose properties are helpful to a dry skin if yours is oily!

Should you wish to ingest any carrier oil helpful to your condition, try them in a salad dressing (see page 254) (not in cooking, as some of the properties are destroyed by strong heat) or take a teaspoonful three times a day if, like me, you can swallow them on their own.

Externally, the oils have an effect on a number of skin problems and for these, the most beneficial carrier oil can be selected. The more severe the problem, the higher should be the percentage of special oil in your mix, to enhance the effects of the essential oils.

Last year, when visiting a supplier from whom we buy cold pressed oils, I smelled and tasted each oil they stocked and was impressed by the different aromas and flavours. In the first edition of my book, *Practical Aromatherapy*, I said that a carrier oil should have little or no odour; at the time I had neither the in-depth knowledge nor the first hand experience I now have. The aromas of carrier oils are, in any case, subtle enough to ensure that the added essential oils will win through!

The stability of a vegetable oil depends on its fatty acid content; those high in saturated fatty acids (SFAs) are more stable than those high in unsaturated fatty acids (UFAs). Stability also depends on the vitamin E content, those vegetable oils containing both SFAs and vitamin E having a longer shelf life.

A number of vegetable oils, such as avocado, sesame, sunflower and wheatgerm contain a variety of minerals which may be impoverished by the use of pesticides and fertilizers during their growing period. Furthermore, molecules from some of these chemicals may permeate into the finished cold pressed product.

With increasing interest in organic plants for drying, or essential oil extraction, an interesting aspect arises. Some aromatherapists go out of their way to buy organic (or naturally grown) essential oils, yet happily dilute these in cold pressed vegetable oils which form about 95 per cent of the final mix yet are *not* organically grown! Organic vegetable oils are quite rare, though fortunately our suppliers abroad cold press their own organically grown seeds and nuts.

Maceration

There are a few plants which contain very interesting properties, but whose essential oils are too difficult or too expensive to distil. In order to benefit from these properties, such plants are chopped up and put into a vat of vegetable oil (usually olive or sunflower) and agitated for several days – the process is called maceration. The vegetable oil acts as a solvent, drawing from the plant any molecules which are soluble in vegetable oil. As we know that essential oils are soluble in vegetable oil, the properties extracted from the plant material include these molecules as well as larger molecules such as plant colouring. The resulting liquid is then filtered and bottled.

Macerated oils include calendula, carrot, hypericum, lime blossom and melissa, but any medicinal plant can be macerated.

If you have a medicinal plant in your garden (or one that is purely aromatic), you can carry out the process described above – on a much smaller scale, of course! The result will be a ready-to-use massage oil containing the properties from the plant you have chosen.

Half-fill a screwtop glass jar with chopped-up plant material. Fill the jar with warm vegetable oil (containing 10 per cent wheatgerm oil to help preserve the end product) and put in a warm place for a week to 10 days, shaking the jar from time to time. Filter off the plant material.

Carrier Oils used in Aromatherapy

Almond Oil, Sweet (Prunus amygdalis var. dulcis)

The sweet almond tree yields a fixed oil obtained by cold pressing. There exists an *essential* oil from bitter almonds, never used in aromatherapy, because of the risk of prussic acid forming during distillation.

Properties and Effects Sweet almond oil contains vitamins A, B_1, B_2 and B_6 and has a high percentage of mono- and polyunsaturated fatty acids. Because it has a small amount of vitamin E, it keeps reasonably well. It protects and softens the skin, soothes inflammation[119] and calms the irritation caused by eczema.

Apricot Kernel Oil *(Prunus armeniaca)*

Apricot, peach and sweet almond yield almost the same oils chemically (therefore having similar effects). Apricot and peach are usually more expensive as they are not produced in such great quantity. Occasionally, almond oil is sold as apricot or peach, so be sure your supplier knows the source of his oil.

Avocado Oil *(Persea americana)*

Avocado oil is pressed from the dried and sliced flesh from fruits which are not good enough for marketing as fresh produce. Being quite a difficult oil to press, it sometimes has a cloudy appearance – even a bit sludgy at the bottom. This should be regarded as a good sign and not a fault, as it indicates that the oil has not been refined. Refined avocado oil is always pale yellow and lacks the rich green colour of the cold pressed oil.

Avocado oil has excellent keeping qualities because of an inbuilt anti-oxidant system, but if chilled (or during the winter), some components are precipitated, causing it to go cloudy. This can be rectified by placing the bottle in a warm place, when the oil will soon return unharmed to normal.

Properties and Effects   Avocado contains both saturated and monoun-saturated fatty acids and vitamins (A, B and D) and is rich in lecithin. It is thought that despite its viscosity, avocado has the ability to penetrate the upper layers of the skin.

Avocado is valuable to the aromatherapist on account of its beneficial effect on dry skin and wrinkles, and it can form up to 25 per cent of the total mix. It is sometimes used in sun preparations on account of its emollient properties and is said to have skin healing properties.[119]

Calendula Oil *(Calendula officinalis)* Macerated Oil

Although sold as a fixed oil, the calendula grown in Europe for medicinal purposes, does not produce any fixed oil itself. The flowerheads contain too little essential oil to make distillation commercially viable, so all active therapeutic properties are usually extracted by maceration (see section at the beginning of the chapter).

Properties and Effects   Calendula oil has anti-inflammatory, anti-spasmodic, choleretic (increasing bile production) and vulnerary (helps healing of wounds) properties, rendering it effective on bed sores, broken

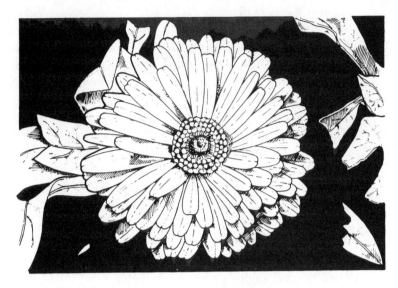

FIGURE 8.1: Calendula

veins, bruises, gum inflammations (and tooth extraction cavities), persistent ulcers, stubborn wounds and varicose veins.[120] It is extremely effective on skin problems; rashes, and in particular, chapped and cracked skin,[121] which makes it an excellent base oil to use when treating dry eczema. N.B. Hypericum and calendula make an excellent synergistic mix to which essential oils can be added.

Although extremely beneficial on its own, the effects are enhanced when essential oils for the condition being treated are added to it. If adding 25 per cent or less of calendula to a basic carrier oil, the addition of the extra essential oils becomes more important.

Carrot Oil *(Daucus carota)* Macerated Oil

True fixed oil of carrot is extracted by maceration (see section on maceration earlier in the chapter) of the finely chopped traditional orange carrot root in a vegetable oil and is rich in beta-carotene. Each time we take our study group to France, we visit the factory which supplies us with macerated organic oils, to watch the maceration process.

I said 'true' fixed oil of carrot, because there is an oil used extensively in the cosmetic industry called carrot oil, that has never seen a carrot! The African marigold (tagetes) is also rich in beta-carotene and this 'carrot' oil is made by adding the beta-carotene extracted from tagetes to a base oil such as soya or sunflower. It has similar properties to true carrot, but the oil is extremely concentrated, with a deeper colour and is not suitable for aromatherapy treatments because of the strong colour.

One of my therapists had a client wanting carrot oil in her treatment mix. Knowing we did not stock it at the time, she bought some from another source. She and the client were concerned to find that, not only was the client orange afterwards, but so were the towels and couch cover! Obviously, the therapist had been given carrot oil made from tagetes! This oil may be therapeutic, but I am sorry it is given such a misleading name – perhaps it is short for carotene oil!

Both tagetes flowers and carrot seeds yield essential oils (see chapter 4).

Properties and Effects   True carrot oil is rich in beta-carotene, vitamins A, B, C, D and E, and essential fatty acids.[122]

Useful on burns, carrot oil is anti-inflammatory. It is known to be an effective rejuvenator, delaying the ageing process, with repeated use. It is therefore a useful ingredient in skin creams or oils which are used every day.

Caution   There are no contra-indications to the use of carrot oil, but excessive ingestion of carrots themselves, or juice, can cause hypervitaminosis (the palms of the hands and soles of the feet become orange and the body skin dry and flaky, taking on an orangey, suntanned look). If these symptoms are ignored, the whole system becomes toxic, causing death in extreme cases.

Coconut Oil (Cocos nucifera)

Coconut oil does not occur naturally, the white flesh, when pressed yielding an odorous solid *fat* which contains therapeutic properties. To obtain coconut oil the fat is subjected to heat (as in hot extraction) and the top, liquid fraction removed. This is usually deodorized for use in both the food and cosmetic industries, as its natural odour is overpowering even with the addition of essential oils. Being a fractionated oil, its use in aromatherapy, where we insist on everything being complete and whole, must be questioned.

Properties and Effects   Coconut oil aids tanning and is reputed to help filter the sun's rays; it is emollient on hair and skin. However, on some people, it can cause an allergic reaction[123] – perhaps because it is not a complete product.

Corn Oil *(Zea mays)*

This oil is produced exclusively by hot extraction (the corn germ containing very little oil) – it is therefore not one of the preferred oils for aromatherapy.

Evening Primrose Oil *(Oenothera biennis)*

Rich in linoleic acid, a polyunsaturated fatty acid, and containing a small percentage of gamma linolenic acid (GLA – known to reduce blood cholesterol),[124] evening primrose oil is extremely useful for the prevention of heart disease. These essential fatty acids are vital for cell and body function and cannot be made by the body itself.

Properties and Effects   Taken internally, evening primrose oil is said to be invaluable for reducing blood pressure, controlling arthritis, relieving eczema, helping schizophrenia and PMS and decreasing hyperactivity in children.[125] However, it has been found that the doses usually prescribed are probably too low to have a noticeable and lasting effect.

Used externally, the oil is helpful for psoriasis, dry, scaly skin and dandruff.[126] It accelerates wound healing and can also be used on eczema.

Grapeseed Oil *(Vitis vinifera)*

Like corn oil, grapeseed oil is produced by hot extraction; it has only about 12 per cent of oil in the seeds.

Life is a series of lessons, and I learned this one in 1990. Since then I have been wondering if grapeseed oil is good enough for aromatherapy. The oil can be 'rescued' after steam extraction (before passing through the refining process) but the extra labour and time involved increases the price substantially.

Properties and Effects   Grapeseed oil contains a high percentage of linoleic acid and some vitamin E and is one of the few oils which is cholesterol-free and easily digested.

It is a gentle emollient, leaving the skin with a satin finish without feeling greasy. It has no known contra-indications and is non-toxic.[127]

Hazelnut Oil *(Corylus avellana)*

Both male and female flowers are present on each hazelnut tree, the nuts yielding an amber yellow oil with a pleasant aroma and a slight flavour of marzipan.

Properties and Effects   Oleic acid (a monounsaturated fatty acid) is the principal constituent, with a small proportion of linoleic acid (a polyunsaturated fatty acid) also being present.

Hazelnut oil is said to penetrate the top layer of the skin slightly, being beneficial for oily or combination skins and effective on acne.[128] It is stimulating to the circulation and also has astringent properties. It may be more economic if required for regular use, to use it in conjunction with a less expensive base oil. However, when using it to benefit skin disorders, it should be used alone as the base, with added essential oils.

As it has been shown to be effective in filtering out some of the harmful rays of the sun (factor equivalent to 10)[129] it can be used in sun lotions.

Hypericum *(Hypericum perforatum)* Macerated Oil

St John's Wort (the common name for hypericum) is another macerated oil (see section on maceration earlier in the chapter). The properties are extracted from the plant when there are plenty of buds present; these give the oil its rich ruby colour (if you press a bud between your fingers they will become red). The open yellow flowers contain no red colour, but tiny black dots on the edges of the petals contain hypericin[130] and a minute amount of essential oil can be obtained from the tiny visible glands on the leaves.

Properties and Effects   An anti-inflammatory oil, hypericum is particularly soothing to inflamed nerves, making it helpful for cases of neuralgia, sciatica and fibrositis. It is indicated on wounds where there is nerve tissue damage and is effective on sprains, burns and bruises.[131] As with calendula, the addition of essential oils increases the therapeutic effects and the two carrier oils together make it even more effective.

Jojoba Oil *(Simmondsia chinensis)*

Jojoba (pronounced 'hohoba') is not an oil but a liquid *wax*, which replaced sperm whale oil in the cosmetics industry when the whale became an endangered species. It is an environmental aid, as planting it saves arid land from becoming desert – plantations cover around 40,000 acres in the United States. It can be used instead of beeswax as an emulsifier in creams.

Jojoba is very stable, having extremely good keeping qualities – it is a pity that it is one of the more expensive oils.

Properties and Effects   The chemical structure of jojoba not only resembles sebum, but the latter can dissolve in it, which makes it a useful oil in cases of acne. The fact that it is also indicated for dry scalp and skin, psoriasis, eczema, sunburn and nappy rash[132] shows it to be a very balancing oil. Jojoba contains an acid (myristic acid) which has anti-inflammatory properties, helpful when mixing a blend for rheumatism and arthritis.

Lime Blossom Oil *(Tilia europaea)* Macerated Oil

The blossoms from this beautiful tree are used mainly in the production of tea (very popular in France), although a small quantity is macerated to produce an oil which is useful to aromatherapists.

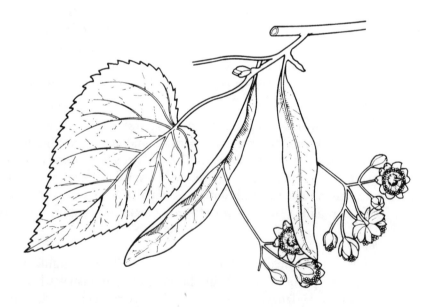

FIGURE 8.2: Lime blossom

Properties and Effects An effective oil to fight the age-old problem of wrinkles, lime blossom oil soothes rheumatic pain and is relaxing, aiding sleep.[133]

Macadamia Oil (Macadamia integrifolia and M. ternifolia)

A fairly new arrival on the aromatherapy scene is the oil from the macadamia nut, grown in New South Wales and Queensland. It is high in palmitoleic acid, a monounsaturated fatty acid that does not occur in any other plant oil but is found in sebum. Fairly stable, the unrefined oil is a soft golden colour with a lovely texture and 'feel' to it and has a hint of an aroma (the refined oil is pale yellow, with no smell).

Properties and Effects Palmitoleic acid in sebum diminishes progressively as we get older and macadamia oil may help replenish this in older skin (perhaps it is more effective internally?) It is highly emollient and its anti-ageing properties are very interesting! Nourishing to a dry and/or mature skin, it has been found useful in sun preparations – it is used in France as an aid against sunburn.

When taken internally it is an effective laxative.

Melissa Oil (Melissa officinalis) Macerated Oil

Macerated melissa oil is only produced in regions where melissa is grown for distillation and tea production. Our supplier produces this from organically grown plants.

Properties and Effects Melissa oil is indicated for massage on 'heavy legs' (fluid retention), especially in combination with cypress essential oil. It is also beneficial on dry and mature skins.

Mullein Flower Oil (Verbascum thapsus) Macerated Oil

A tall plant, whose common name is Aaron's rod, mullein has a crop of yellow flowers on a long head and grows wild by the roadside. The oil is macerated in the south of France.

Properties and Effects Mullein oil is antiseptic, softening to the skin and soothing to rheumatic inflammation and neuralgia. It is useful against haemorrhoids, wounds and chilblains.[133]

Olive Oil *(Olea europaea)*

Traditionally used for centuries in cooking and healing, virgin pressed olive oil is popular on supermarket shelves because of its monounsaturated fatty acid content, effective in the prevention of high cholesterol and heart disease, as well as its wonderful flavour. Its green colour is due to a small percentage of chlorophyll in the flesh, from which the oil is taken, and it is an ideal cooking oil for health conscious people.

Properties and Effects   Externally olive oil is emollient, soothing to inflamed skin and good for sprains and bruises. It is a little heavy for massage but can be added 50/50 to a less viscous oil.

When ingested, it is not only prophylactic against heart disease, but is a help against hyperacidity and constipation.

Peach Kernel Oil *(Prunus persica)*

See Apricot Kernel Oil.

Peanut Oil *(Arachis hypogaea)*

Peanut oil is a less stable oil regarding keeping qualities and has quite a noticeable aroma (not unpleasant and not so strong as coconut). It is mostly available only in the refined state although a small quantity is cold pressed in France.

Properties and Effects   An emollient oil (particularly for arthritis and sunburn), peanut, rather oily to use on its own for massage, is perfectly acceptable for self-application to specific areas or to blend with another less viscous carrier oil. However, people with nut allergies should avoid peanut in particular.[134]

Rose Hip Oil *(Rosa canina, R. mollis)*

Coming mostly from wild plants, this oil is usually organic and yields a lovely golden red oil, often obtained, unfortunately, by solvent extraction.

Properties and Effects   Research in Chile shows rose hip oil to be a tissue regenerator (perhaps due to its high unsaturated fatty acid content), making it an excellent oil for a mature skin. It has been shown to be effective on scars, wounds, burns (including sunburn), eczema and ageing and I am surprised it is not used more universally.

Safflower Oil *(Carthamus tinctorius)*

Safflower, like sunflower, belongs to the Compositae family and has an orangey yellow flower. Safflower seeds were discovered in 3,000-year-old Egyptian tombs and both flowers and seeds have been used in the past as a dye.

Properties and Effects   Yet another oil high in polyunsaturated fatty acids, safflower oil helps a number of circulatory problems and, taken internally, is said to be helpful for bronchial asthma. It is beneficial on painful, inflamed joints, sprains and bruises. It is one of the less stable oils (except when it is refined, when it has preservatives added to it).

Sesame Oil *(Sesamum indicum)*

The seeds of the sesame plant are contained inside a long nut and give a high yield of clear pale yellow oil when cold pressed.

Properties and Effects   The pressed oil is rich in vitamins and minerals, its vitamin E and sesamol content giving the oil excellent stability.

It is beneficial for dry skin, psoriasis and eczema[135] and protects the skin to a certain extent from the harmful rays of the sun.

Soya Bean Oil *(Glycine soja)*

Soya bean oil is usually obtained by solvent extraction, as the beans have a low oil content. Although containing some vitamin C, it is not as rich a source as sunflower or wheatgerm oils. Prone to oxidation, it can be a sensitizer (see chapter 6), so it may be wise not to use it in aromatherapy.

Sunflower Oil *(Helianthus annuus)*

Although most sunflower oil is solvent extracted, you can obtain an oil from organically grown plants that is cold pressed. This oil has a lovely light texture and is very pleasant to use, leaving the skin with a satin-smooth, non-greasy feel – a good substitute for grapeseed!

Properties and Effects   Sunflower oil contains vitamins A, B, D and E (the principal one) and is high in unsaturated fatty acids, making it helpful against arteriosclerosis. It has a prophylactic effect on the skin and is beneficial to leg ulcers, bruises and skin diseases. Sunflower oil has diuretic properties, is expectorant and as it contains inulin, it is useful in the treatment of asthma.[136]

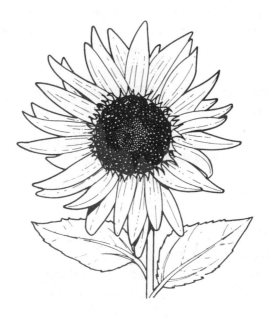

FIGURE 8.3: Sunflower

The leaves and flowers have been used in Russia for years against chest problems such as bronchitis.

Wheatgerm Oil *(Triticum vulgare)*

Wheatgerm oil is a rich orangey brown colour and, due to its high vitamin E content, is widely used to increase the keeping qualities of less stable oils – a minimum of 5–10 per cent should be added to the base oil, up to 20 per cent if the oil has low stability.

Properties and Effects   Wheatgerm is useful on dry and mature skins,[137] though too heavy to use by itself for massage.

Taken internally, it is said to help prevent varicose veins, eczema and indigestion and helps to remove cholesterol deposits from the arteries.

Caution   As it is from a protein, it could be contra-indicated for anyone prone to allergies. If you are not sure, test it first (see chapter 6).

TABLE 5: Beneficial Properties of some Fixed and Macerated Vegetable Oils

	Avocado	Calendula*	Carrot*	Evening primrose	Hazelnut	Hypericum*	Jojoba	Lime blossom*	Macadamia	Melissa*	Mullein*	Olive	Peanut	Rose hip	Safflower	Sesame	Sunflower	Wheatgerm
Acne					X		X											
Bed sores		X																
Broken veins		X									X							
Bruises		X				X						X			X		X	
Burns			X			X								X				
Chapped skin		X																
Chilblains											X							
Dandruff				X														
Dry scalp				X			X											
Dry skin	X			X		X			X	X						X		X
Eczema		X		X		X								X		X		
Fibrositis						X												
Fluid retention										X								
Haemorrhoids											X							
Inflammation		X	X			X	X					X			X			
Mature skin			X						X	X				X				X
Nappy rash		X	X			X								X		X		
Neuralgia						X					X							
Oily skin				X		X												
Psoriasis						X									X			
Rejuvenating			X					X						X				
Relaxing (sleep)								X										
Rheumatism/Arthritis						X		X			X		X					
Scars														X				
Sciatica						X												
Skin rashes		X				X												
Sprains												X			X			
Sunburn	X	X	X			X		X			X	X	X					
Sun protection	X								X							X		
Ulcers		X															X	
Varicose veins		X									X							
Wounds											X			X				
Wrinkles	X							X	X					X				

* Macerated oils

9 *The Holistic Approach*

There are two concepts of medicine which are complementary to, rather than in disagreement with, one another. Orthodox and natural medicine are head and tail of the same coin; it is a twin situation and genuine co-operation and mutual respect are the overall aim.[138] Orthodox medicine (allopathy), often referred to as classical medicine, looks on sickness as 'accidental' – a combination of signals and symptoms due to an exterior damaging agent. As classical medicine advanced through the ages these exterior agents have been given various names – 'a spirit' or 'bad luck' and eventually, as knowledge increased, 'microbe', 'bacteria', 'virus', etc. Classical medicine tries to eliminate these in order to heal the patient.

In the 1960s and 70s, when words like 'peace', 'love', 'ecology' and 'organic' were making inroads, practitioners of other, natural, forms of medicine made their appearance. We called them alternative (not such a good word), complementary (much better!), natural, parallel (in France), or energetic medicine. Complementary therapies try to treat the whole person and help us to adapt to our surroundings (climate, food, stress) and to live harmoniously with ourselves and others. Illness in these circumstances is usually the result of poor adaptation to the environment, and complementary therapists aim to help people to adjust their lifestyle, rather than help them to suppress symptoms.

Natural therapies have become known as 'listening therapies' where practitioners try to discover the reason behind the body's cry for help, which manifests itself in the form of headaches, stomach upsets, breathing problems, etc. For example, if a person suffers from repeated attacks of gastroenteritis, classical medicine will look at the possibility of intrusion by a microbe or bacteria and give the appropriate counter-agent – probably an antibiotic (which means 'against life'). This will probably rid the body of the symptoms, but as it is unable to distinguish between good and bad bacteria, the good bacteria needed by the patient in order to function well are also killed.[139] Sometimes, with repeated treatment by antibiotics, either the immune system is impoverished, opening the body to further infection, or the body builds up a resistance to that particular antibiotic agent, which no longer has an effect on the symptoms presented.

A complementary therapist, however, would see the symptoms in the light of the whole being – as clues to the real disease/imbalance. He or she may suggest that the reason the unwanted bacteria were able to penetrate the intestine was because that person's defence system was not strong enough to fight off the invaders. The gastroenteritis may be due to a weakness in the liver or kidneys, the type of food eaten, allergens, or an emotional situation. The whole organism would be studied in relation to the person's environment and lifestyle, and the advice and treatment given would take these elements into account.

The essential oils chosen for aromatherapy treatment may be stress-relieving or kidney-strengthening, as well as antibacterial, depending on the person's needs. Bactericidal essential oils are, to some extent, probiotic (which means 'for life') so only the unwanted bacteria are eliminated, without harming those necessary for life.

After diet and lifestyle advice has been given, the following essential oils may be chosen, those suggested being also stress-relieving, should this be partly responsible for the condition:

Sweet thyme and bergamot to strengthen the immune system (sweet thyme, especially the geraniol chemotype is an excellent bactericide[140] and bergamot is antispasmodic to the intestines).
Sandalwood and/or juniper to strengthen the kidneys.[141]
Basil as a nerve tonic.[142]

The aromatherapy treatment advised may include some of the following.

A back and abdominal massage, if it were felt that an initial boost to the system was needed.
A Swiss reflex treatment on the feet, using the same essential oils in a cream base, with instructions on how to continue this at home.
An oil or lotion, containing five drops each of sweet thyme, bergamot and

basil to be applied to the abdomen and small of the back half an hour before meals.

The same essential oils (two drops of each to be used without a carrier) for inhalation four or five times a day or to put in the bath.

An abdominal compress (two drops each of the three essential oils in ¼–½ pint of warm water) before retiring at night.

A tea (as described in chapter 7) using two drops of sweet thyme and one drop each of bergamot and sandalwood in 1 litre/1½ pints water, drinking one cup half an hour before meals.

This 'case' may serve to illustrate that an aromatherapy treatment does not always include a full body massage; not everyone enjoys being massaged and some people may prefer to have advice on how to care for their imbalance in the privacy of their own home.

Nevertheless, where stress and depression are a major cause of a health imbalance, then, in my opinion, a full aromatherapy body massage is the best complementary therapy treatment available. It is also an excellent prophylactic treatment to ensure continuation of good health.

The age of complementary therapies is advancing quickly. Why? Possibly because the emphasis on healing has been switched from treating the physical aspect of disease with chemical drugs (which sometimes merely treat, or suppress, the symptoms), to treating the whole person, physical, mental and spiritual, aided by natural medicines and correct eating habits. The holistic approach is to look for the underlying cause of the disease, and to treat this rather than the symptoms. The cause may lie in any of several different aspects of the patient's lifestyle.

Emotional Lifestyle

Much more emphasis is placed nowadays on the relationship between our health and our emotional state. Psychoneuroimmunology, a fairly new discipline, is the study of how thoughts can influence the brain and directly affect the health of cells in all parts of the body – and indeed, one's whole outlook on life. The subject is now being introduced into the syllabus at some medical colleges as the truth of this becomes more and more apparent. There is still a lot of work to be done on the subject as, although the pathways between the brain and the immune system are known to be there, evidence of how they operate is difficult to pin down, since different individuals react in different ways to the same stimulus (the placebo group in a clinical test often produces better results than the one given the medicine!)

> 'In research it has now been shown that dummy painkillers are 56 per cent as effective in killing chronic pain as morphine, one of the most powerful of all painkilling drugs.'[143]

We must all agree to a certain extent with the saying 'we are what we eat'. Without going into psychoneuroimmunology too deeply (the subject deserves a whole book devoted to it), its philosophy is that 'we are what we think'. Happy, positive thoughts exert a positive influence on both health and life in general, whereas negative emotions are self-inflicted wounds which effectively close down the immune system, leaving the body vulnerable to a wide range of disease processes.[144]

> 'the depression of the spirits at these melancholy occasions [funerals] ... disposes them to some of the worst effects of the chills.'[144]

Those who are continually discontented, critical of self and others (or displaying other negative emotions) are the very ones who may attract illness and personal disasters. Conversely, how many really happy, contented people are continually ill?

> 'Many disorders such as digestive ulcers, colitis, hypertension, asthma, are either directly caused by emotional/mental processes or at the very least are significantly exacerbated by them.'[145]

One thing is certain – smiling and laughing have a positive effect on health, even if the smiling is forced (true!) If ever I feel 'down' or have a headache coming on (neither happens often!) I force my mouth into a smile and begin to feel better almost immediately (nine times out of ten I do not even have to reach for my essential oils). Reading the following two snippets somewhere introduced me to the art:

'Californian Norman Cousins, diagnosed as having a chronic degenerative illness, shut himself up with a pile of Charlie Chaplin videos and laughed himself back to health.'

'Michigan psychologist Robert Zajonc says that faking smiling still triggers a reaction in your brain, making you feel happier and healthier. It is hard to feel stressed when you are beaming – even artificially!'

I say try it too! You have nothing to lose but your illness or unhappiness.

'A merry heart doeth good like a medicine; but a broken spirit drieth the bones.'

Proverbs 17:22

The effect which thoughts can have on life has been proved by people who have either tried positive thinking, mind dynamics or visualization, or put their whole faith and trust in God. Cancers have been healed, situations changed for the better, success ensured – all through positive application of the mind, which influences the emotions, which in turn influence health and life.

Mental attitudes play a far greater part in day-to-day health than is realized. It is not always easy to change to a positive attitude when suffering, but those who can, have recovered even from terminal diseases like cancer. My gentle, lovable mother, crippled with chronic arthritis from the age of 33 (and on cortisone tablets for 29 years – with all their horrific side effects), sadly found it impossible to believe it could be done, but fortunately I was able to apply it to myself. Having been told that arthritis was hereditary, I was 'waiting' for myself to contract the disease around the age of 33 (my bone structure and physical attributes are very similar to my mother's). At 35 my index finger and thumb muscles began to ache regularly. My other fingers gradually became misshapen and stiff, reducing my ability to grip things well – exactly how my mother's disease started!

Fortunately for me, at the age of 40 I attended a 'Mind Dynamics' course (this is another story!) which changed my life, in more ways than one. We were taught visualization among other things, and I told my fingers I was not going to have arthritis – so there! I told them daily; I visualized myself pain-free and healthy and before long I realized I had been pain-free for ages! Twenty years later I still do not have arthritis (or any pain), though my joints have retained their funny shape!

For those who find positive thinking difficult, or cannot have faith strong enough to believe that things can be changed, essential oils are an alternative route. For those who really try to achieve their aim, it will widen that route into a motorway!

Essential oils affect our health from the same starting point as our thoughts – the mind and emotions. This time it is the chemicals in the essential oils which are responsible for influencing the brain (chapter 7) to our good. Their action may give a purely emotional result, i.e. the relief of stress (due to anger, hate, greed, jealousy, pressure of work, insensitivity to others, etc.) or depression (due to fear, loneliness, melancholy, grief, mourning, lack of self-confidence, etc.), but the relief of the stressful or depressive state automatically, as in the psychoneuroimmunology theory, sets the healing process in motion, relieving any physical problems which may have been the result.

Although you may know your ill health is possibly based on stress or depression, always search diligently to see if there is a further emotional cause. Maybe you have always bottled up your emotions, never letting people see how you really feel; perhaps you have continuously been jealous of people who have better luck, more money, a nicer figure, more skilful or amusing conversational powers than you have? Think carefully . . . there is always a reason for a long standing illness, and it may happen to be an emotional one. Maybe you were once hurt at a new school by children who made fun of the accent you brought with you from another area; maybe you subconsciously nurtured the anger you felt when your parents were always quarrelling – there just may be an emotional reason for your ill health.

We may, in all probability, neither like nor want to believe the reason when, or if, we find one. Be that as it may, when selecting essential oils, decide at least whether your problem is based on stress or depression. If you believe there may be another emotional reason, get to work with positive thinking to negate it. List all the oils you can find which may help your emotional state, following this by listing essential oils which will help the symptoms you are suffering (see Table 6 in this chapter and the Therapeutic Effects list in chapter 14). You will be sure to find at least two or three which appear on both lists and these are the ones to use first.

TABLE 6: Therapeutic Effects of Oils on Emotional Symptoms

	Basil (Ocimum basilicum)	Bergamot (Citrus bergamia)	Cedarwood (Cedrus atlantica)	R. Chamomile (Chamaemelum nobile)	Clary (Salvia sclarea)	Coriander (Coriandrum sativum)	Cypress (Cupressus sempervirens)	Eucalyptus (Eucalyptus smithii)	Frankincense (Boswellia carteri)	Geranium (Pelargonium graveolens)	Ginger (Zingiber officinale)	Juniperberry (Juniperus communis)	Lavender (Lavandula angustifolia)
Agitation	X	X		X	X	X			X	X		X	X
Anger	X	X		X		X	X		X	X		X	X
Apathy	X	X		X	X	X			X	X	X	X	
Argumentativeness					X			X				X	
Boredom	X		X	X	X				X		X		
Confusion	X	X	X	X	X		X	X	X	X		X	X
Daydreaming					X	X	X	X	X			X	X
Despair			X		X				X	X			
Despondency	X				X	X			X		X		
Disappointment					X			X	X		X	X	
Discouragement		X	X		X				X			X	X
Fear	X	X		X	X	X			X	X	X	X	X
Forgetfulness	X		X	X		X		X					
Frustration				X	X		X		X			X	X
Grief (sorrow)	X	X			X	X		X	X			X	X
Guilt	X			X	X		X	X	X	X		X	X
Irritability		X		X	X	X	X		X	X		X	X
Jealousy	X	X			X			X		X		X	X
Lethargy	X	X	X	X						X	X	X	
Mood swings		X			X	X	X			X	X	X	X
Nightmares	X	X			X	X							X
Obsession				X	X		X	X		X			X
Panic	X	X		X	X				X				X
Poor concentration	X		X			X	X	X				X	X
Resentment				X	X								X
Restlessness		X	X	X	X			X			X	X	X
Shock					X								
Timidity	X		X		X	X			X			X	X

Lemon (Citrus limon)	Mandarin (Citrus reticulata)	Marjoram, sweet (Origanum majorana)	Melissa, true (Melissa officinalis)	Myrrh (Commiphora myrrha)	Neroli (Citrus aurantium v. amara)	Niaouli (Melaleuca viridiflora)	Orange, bitter (Citrus aurantium v. amara)	Peppermint (Mentha x piperita)	Petitgrain (Citrus aurantium v. amara)	Rose otto (Rosa centifolia)	Rosemary (Rosmarinus officinalis)	Rosewood (Aniba rosaeodora)	Sandalwood (Santalum album)	Thyme, sweet (Thymus vulgaris)	Ylang ylang (Cananga odorata)
	X	X	X	X			X	X	X	X			X	X	X
X	X	X	X	X		X	X	X	X	X	X		X	X	X
X		X			X	X	X	X			X			X	X
	X					X	X		X		X			X	X
	X	X					X	X			X			X	X
		X			X	X			X		X	X	X	X	X
X					X	X	X	X	X	X		X	X	X	X
		X	X		X						X		X	X	X
		X			X	X		X	X			X	X	X	X
		X			X	X				X	X			X	X
		X	X		X			X		X	X		X	X	X
		X	X	X		X	X	X		X	X		X	X	X
X	X						X	X			X			X	X
X	X					X	X	X						X	X
		X	X		X	X	X	X	X	X	X	X		X	
		X								X	X		X	X	
X	X	X	X	X		X	X	X	X	X			X	X	X
X						X	X	X		X	X	X	X	X	X
X	X	X			X		X			X	X		X	X	X
		X				X			X	X	X	X	X	X	X
X	X	X	X	X			X						X		X
X	X	X	X					X	X	X			X		X
		X		X	X		X			X	X		X	X	X
X		X					X	X			X			X	
X		X									X			X	
	X		X	X	X		X		X		X				X
		X		X	X				X						X
X		X			X		X						X	X	X

The volatility of an essential oil can play a big part in its emotional effects (see chapter 3).

Top notes, because they are usually the most volatile, are indicated when the mind needs a lift, as in poor concentration or despondency. Base notes, being more relaxing, usually come into their own for relieving intense feelings which are difficult to let go – anxieties and stresses, such as grief or panic or fear – bringing a more secure or 'grounded' feeling. Middle notes are balancing, so may be indicated for mood swings and confusion.

However, neither emotions nor essential oils are as simple as that and you may find that an oil from another note may be helpful to you. It is therefore always best to select an oil from each volatility range (or at least from two) as you may need both the energizing *and* the calming effects or perhaps the calming and balancing ones, or even all three! When making your choice, try to achieve an aesthetically pleasing aroma as well as a therapeutically effective blend; the fact that you love the smell is healing in itself. Don't forget to write down all your blends on a notepad, and keep it with your essential oils.

Nutritional Lifestyle

We said at the beginning of this chapter that 'we are what we eat'. If you cannot find an emotional cause for your problem, have a look at your diet – your nutritional lifestyle. The cause of your condition could be due to incorrect eating habits. There is an abundant variety of food available nowadays but little is naturally rich in nutrients. Many foods are processed, refined and contain additives, colourings and preservatives. This may make shopping and cooking much easier, but can lead to an imbalanced nutrient intake. At one time a rich meal like Christmas dinner was a real treat; now cookery books and restaurants vie with each other to give us sumptuous sauces and unusual meals, and continual adverts on television tempt us to eat more foods containing refined sugars and starches. Our digestive systems find this difficult to cope with on a regular basis, and as a result our health begins to suffer, becoming worse unless the food pattern is altered. There is no need to make a radical change to vegan or macrobiotic overnight – this will not help your digestive system at all. A **gradual** cutting out of poor quality foods, introducing those of high nutritional value, will be far better for your health.

Shops and supermarkets devote about four-fifths of their shelf space to tinned or pre-prepared foods, which are either lacking in (or have added to them artificially) the nutrients on which our digestive systems normally work to the benefit of our health. Tasteless (but beautiful looking) fruits and vegetables, grown with chemicals to yield a uniform size and a greater yield per plant, are everywhere. I suppose it is all in the name of 'progress' and 'no time to cook'.

Healthy Rations

Fresh fruits and vegetables give us in natural form the vitamins and minerals that are needed to keep the human body in optimum condition.

Health is a complex subject and it does not necessarily follow that because there is absence of disease one is in good health. Neither does having an acute illness mean that vitality and strength arc not present – a strong, healthy body efficiently throws off an acute illness with very little help because it is self-regulating and self-healing.

Even in wartime, when food was rationed, the health of the nation as a whole did not suffer – in fact, there is more ill health nowadays as a result of too much food than there was then with rationing! The reason was no doubt because sweets and chocolate were rationed and the quality of the food available was very much better – large scale farming methods and use of refined foods, etc. had not yet made their big entrance. With the ingestion of whole, untampered-with, nutritious food the body had everything it needed, extra nutrients in the form of tablets not being necessary.

Today, good food alone should still be revitalizing to the system; any discomfort felt after eating, if not due to hasty consumption or insufficient chewing, may be due to the consumption of an unnecessary, though tempting, food item. After a nutritious and healthy salad lunch I always feel satisfied, bright and energetic, and if I have a sweet (which is not often nowadays) I usually regret it.

Dietary Suggestions

Here is one suggestion for preparing salads daily. Cut up into small cubes (¼ inch/½ cm) a selection of seven or eight different vegetables and fruits (shredding cabbage and lettuce finely). Mix them all together with just enough dressing (not salad cream) or plain yogurt, French mustard and hazelnut or walnut oil to moisten when well tossed. You can use lettuce (different kinds); parsley; carrot; radishes; bean sprouts; avocado; apple;

peppers (different colours); cucumber; tomato; peach; plum; pear; nuts; seeds etc. This salad is different every time!

Often there are foods you appear to be able to digest, but which may still be responsible for causing your symptoms. Make sure there is nothing you are eating or drinking which may be contra-indicated for your particular health condition – there are specific foods detrimental to specific conditions, such as orange juice for arthritis and milk for asthma (see Further Reading). There are also general dietary rules to follow which can effect a positive influence on your state of health.

Too much red meat is a strain on the digestive system; twice a week is sufficient for a meat eater. Chicken and other fowl are much easier to digest, as is fish. Alkaline-forming foods are better than acid-forming foods, since a surfeit of acid in the body is the forerunner of disease and if allowed to build up in the reticulo-endothelial system (RES), will, without doubt, result in ill health to some degree or another. If you suffer from any allergic complaint such as asthma, hay fever or eczema, all dairy products should be completely eliminated from your diet (see Chapter 6 – Case Example on eczema). If you are a migraine sufferer, chocolate (even one piece), caffeine (in tea as well as coffee) and (for some people) cheese, can bring on an attack and really should be avoided altogether.

The RES

The reticulo-endothelial system (RES) is made up of cells liberally distributed throughout the whole body. It plays an essential part in immunity to infection. These cells include phagocytes (Greek *phago* = I eat; *kytos* = cell), which can destroy bacteria and are found in the bone marrow, spleen, lymph nodes, liver, kidneys – in fact, everywhere in the body. The system is one of storage, exchange, elimination and defence and deals with the toxins from food, drugs, medicines and negative thoughts (see Figure 9.1). In a healthy, balanced person the RES remains healthy and balanced, but if the system is overloaded or blocked with toxins, the body initiates disease symptoms. Incidentally, the subconscious is the RES of the mind.[145]

If the diet (and/or thoughts) is changed for the better, or medicinal drugs are no longer needed, the healthy cells finding their way into the RES will be exchanged for some of the toxins there; these will be discharged back into the blood supply and eliminated.[146] If eating habits

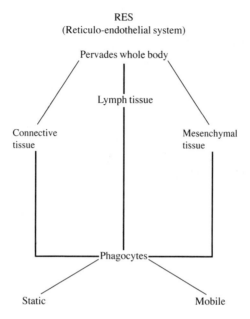

FIGURE 9:1

and thinking are not changed, the system becomes even more blocked, eventually being unable to cope any more. The result is a low energy level, with repetitions of initial symptoms – colds, inflammations, stomach upsets, etc. (see Figure 9.2). This is a warning that the body cannot cope on its own and is now in a sub-acute stage which could gradually become chronic. Attempts to heal at this stage by the repeated use of antibiotics will not be successful (in the first, acute stage, perhaps – but not when the body succumbs again and again). See Figure 9.3. It now becomes a question of building up the immune system so that the body can fight its *own* battle toward better health.

Reversal of this sad state *is* possible, though it needs real and continued effort on the part of the sufferer. See Figure 9.4.

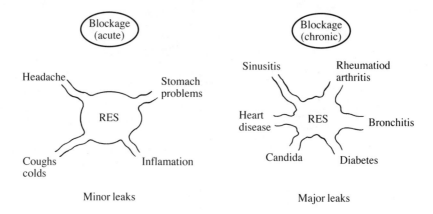

Minor leaks

FIGURE 9.2

Major leaks

FIGURE 9.3

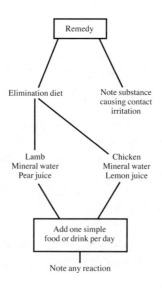

FIGURE 9.4

Exercise Lifestyle

Some people achieve the amount of exercise needed for good health from their normal daily routine. However, if all day is spent sitting at a desk or standing behind a counter, the health may suffer as a result and exercise of some sort may be needed to keep the blood circulation flowing fluently enough to dispose of any toxins waiting to be released. I say exercise of 'some sort', because I am not referring here to exercise for losing weight – but to that which would be considered beneficial to the general health.

The easiest form of exercise is a daily 15-minute brisk walk. This is particularly beneficial for emotional upsets like anger or grief, especially if you live in the country or near a park, where you can turn your thoughts to the wonders of creation, concentrating on the amazing number of variations in the leaves and flowers, the way they are made and the combinations of colours. If you really concentrate on this (and smile!), you will find yourself returning home in a more serene and contented frame of mind.

If a short walk is neither possible nor enjoyed, try going up and down stairs continuously for five minutes. This is an excellent exercise not only for the circulation (and therefore for the general health) but also for varicose veins. If you live in a bungalow, high stepping on the spot or around the dining room table, flexing your feet well, is a reasonable, if strange-looking, alternative!

Another helpful exercise which can be done for a few minutes a number of times during the day, even whilst sitting at a desk or computer, or in another sedentary occupation, is to raise and lower your heels and then your toes firmly, conscious of the flexing and relaxing of the calf muscles – this accelerates the blood flow back to the heart. Blood flowing away from the heart has no problem going downhill, but for the uphill flow back to the heart it needs the help of arm and leg movements. The clenching and unclenching of fists gives blood vessels in the arms considerable help in this direction. These two exercises are invaluable for those whose extremities are always cold and for those with a tendency to varicose veins.

Social Lifestyle

Smoking is on the decrease already among more mature people but is unfortunately on the increase among the young, especially young women, largely due to a sneaky style of advertising. It is now accepted that inhalation of tobacco smoke, whether passive or active, has a detrimental effect on the health. Some people, I agree, seem unaffected by it – we are all individuals, some with stronger lungs than others, and the sad thing is that no-one knows which category they belong to until it is too late! Smoking, once begun, becomes a habit which can be hard to break. If you *want* to break it, it can be done by positive thinking, psychotherapy and even with essential oils. However, if deep down you do not want to give it up, nothing externally can help you. You alone can cure yourself. This also applies to overconsumption of beer, spirits and wine. Drinking one or two glasses of wine a day is good for the health. It is when excess amounts of alcoholic drinks are consumed daily that the liver begins to object to the toxic overload.

If you feel your health problem may be due in part to lack of self-confidence, loneliness or fear, it would help if you could enrol on an evening class or join a theatre or music club, for example (whichever is the easiest for you to summon up the courage to do!) Practise positive thinking and choose essential oils recognized for their ability to give clarity of thought, livening of the spirit and stimulation to the nervous system (basil, bergamot, Roman chamomile, sweet marjoram, rose *otto*).

Everything in this chapter to do with trying to retain, or regain, good health involves *work* on our part – we are responsible for our own health and no-one else can do it for us. Other people can advise and recommend, but only *we* can carry out the advice! In so doing we allow Nature to take its course, and it is Nature that ultimately cures all ills.

> 'Neither (medicine or surgery) can do anything but remove obstructions, neither can cure; nature alone cures. Surgery removes the bullet out of the limb, which is the obstruction to cure, but nature heals the wounds . . . And what nursing has to do in either case is to put the patient in the best condition for nature to act upon him.'
>
> Florence Nightingale

Every disease in the universe can be cured, but not every patient. Some fear change and therefore do not want to be cured. Some *need* illness to engage in life – they like to visit different doctors. Sometimes our job can make us ill; singers of depressing songs and actors continually playing parts such as Macbeth can become ill through repetition of the negative words. Furthermore, there are people who enjoy being 'ill' – they don't really want to be cured. Their ailments bring them sympathy and attention and give them a talking point! Such people are as difficult to help as those who are unable to recognize any long-standing emotional imbalance in themselves; it too, is emotional – a longing for sympathy, recognition or even power – power to disrupt other people's lives.

A personal example illustrates this: Mary, who was interested in aromatherapy for her minor ailments or a relaxing bath, mentioned to me one day that her husband was a chronic asthmatic. Naturally I asked if he had ever used any essential oils. The answer was 'no – he won't try them'. During the conversation that followed it transpired that whenever she wanted to go anywhere other than work, he had an asthma attack, and even the children said he did it on purpose. Mary tried using essential oils in a vaporizer, saying they were for her, and noticed he needed his inhaler less often. Despite the fact that his breathing was definitely easier, her husband said he couldn't stand the smell – it made him feel ill!

There are many stories like this one – if these people *really* wanted to get better, they could do it; the fact is, they are often frightened that they *will* improve! See Figure 9.5.

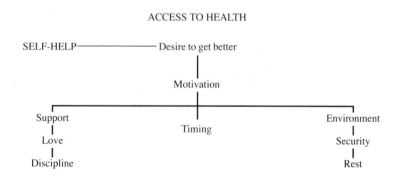

ACCESS TO HEALTH

FIGURE 9:5

Realizing now that some effort is necessary to improve your health, it may be easier to look at one lifestyle at a time. As with slimming, if the effort needed is too much, one soon loses heart and is back on the normal routine. Tackle only what you know you can cope with without this happening. An exercise done for only two minutes, if done every day, will easily become a habit and the time spent on it can then be increased. As far as nutrition is concerned, first remove only one processed or non-nutritious food from your normal diet, replacing it with one beneficial one.

Try visualizing something simple for only two minutes each time you wake up, before getting out of bed (the mind is in a more receptive state at this time of day). If you are trying to cut out smoking, visualize your hand on a packet of cigarettes and draw a big cross over it; see yourself walking past a cigarette counter, turning away your head, refusing an offered cigarette at a party – anything. The important thing is to do whatever you find easiest *every day* until your mind knows you really mean it! If it is overeating to which you have to say goodbye, visualize yourself pushing plates of food away, etc. It can also be done with an emotion; if someone at work makes you feel angry, picture yourself smiling at him or her, physically putting your mouth into the shape of a smile whenever you think of that person – force your mouth into a grin; if you are nervous about joining a club or speaking to your boss, picture yourself doing it for a while – it makes realizing the action so much easier! If you persist each day, and can increase the time spent on visualization and/or prayer (which is visualization with God), you will be able to put all your desires into reality.

Work of whatever nature is always rewarded. Very occasionally we may put in a lot of work and the reward is negative – e.g. you burn your cake or the story you sent to a magazine is not accepted, but the fact remains that there is always a reward and 99 times out of 100, the results are positive.

Practical Application

Looking at life in a truly holistic way, making a list of as many as possible of the facets which may be responsible for your health imbalance, is the first piece of work to be done (see Table 7). Be sure to include all lifestyles, writing them down in separate columns – feelings, diet, exercise (if needed) and socializing. This is your first piece of work.

Now study your columns, writing down underneath the positive thoughts you know would help your situation; the foods you should not be eating and (separately) those essential for your health; the exercises that it would be possible for you to accomplish and which you know would be beneficial; the evening classes, clubs and social events that you would like to go to if you could. Now underline one 'job of work' only, in each column – the execution of these is your 'work' for the next two to four weeks. It is highly unlikely you will fill all five columns, but if you do, leave either the exercises or the social life (whichever is the most difficult for you to achieve) until the next session.

Now for the essential oils to support you in your efforts. On a new sheet list those which will ease your emotional state (see Table 6, page 180), then those which will benefit the symptoms showing themselves (see therapeutic reference list in chapter 14). In the emotional column underline any which appear also in the symptoms column, selecting two, three or four from those which match your most problematic symptom (see Table 8a). Should there not be any which match, choose two from each column. Write down the methods of use, underlining those you would find the easiest to carry out on a regular basis (see Table 8b).

As soon as you have adapted to this new routine, underline one more item from each of the first four columns in a different colour and set to work adding them to your existing 'workload', perhaps, though not necessarily, changing your essential oils as one or two symptoms are relieved. Work at this for the next month, then repeat the underlining to give the increased workload for month three.

You are now well on the way to a holistic health cure – looking at the whole body to pinpoint and eliminate the 'adulterant' toxic factors, nourishing it with whole, unadulterated foods, thinking positive, unadulterated thoughts and using whole, unadulterated essential oils. This will have a positive effect on the whole being. Studying health in this holistic fashion (where symptoms are not suppressed or augmented by drugs) is of paramount importance in order to get the best out of life.

If already on medication from your doctor, do not stop taking your tablets at this stage. If you are on tablets for secondary symptoms, e.g. constipation or insomnia, these symptoms may be relieved first. When you feel you have made some improvement, go to your doctor and ask if you can reduce the dose a little. If you are confident about your improvement (and your doctor is empathetic with complementary medicine), he

TABLE 7: Plan of Action

POSITIVE THOUGHTS	UNHELPFUL FOODS	HEALTHY FOODS	
Tell yourself you feel much better (even if you don't at first!)	All the food and drink which may not be good for your health, e.g.	All the foods you know you should be eating, and which you like, e.g	
Smile a lot	Red meat	Chicken	Trout
Think happy thoughts	Chocolate	Carrots	Cod
Visualize good health	Cow's milk	Leeks	Salmon
etc.	Cola	Cabbage	Wholemeal bread
	Coffee	Turnip	Baked potatoes
	Alcohol	Sprouts	Prunes
	(Cigarettes may also be put here)	Beans	Apples

EXERCISE

Exercises you could do if necessary, e.g.
Daily walk
Stair exercise
Cycling
Tennis
Badminton
etc.

SOCIALIZING

Invite friends round for coffee
Go to the theatre
Join a theatre club
Join a rambling club
etc.

EMOTIONAL OILS

Stress, depression, fear, guilt, anger, etc, e.g.

FRUSTRATION
Roman chamomile√HA.
Cypress√
Frankincense√A
Juniperberry√A
Lemon√HA
Mandarin√C
Bitter orange√C
Sweet thyme√A

IRRITABILITY

Tick oils above where there are any repeats.

Lavender√HA

SYMPTOMATIC OILS

List symptoms, e.g.

Headaches (H)
Constipation (C)
Aching joints (A)

Mark the appropriate oils with first
letter in emotional column on the left.

8b

ESSENTIAL OILS CHOSEN

2 drops Roman chamomile
2 drops lemon
1–2 drops lavender if needed
2 drops bitter orange or mandarin

Roman chamomile and lemon will help the emotions and two of the problems, therefore are the main oils. Bitter orange or mandarin will help the constipation. Lavender can be added, if the aroma needs adjusting, as it helps the headaches, the aching joints and the irritability.

METHODS OF USE

Inhalation   Baths

Compresses   Gargles

Self application   Massage

Professional treatment

or she will be only too pleased for you to try and manage on a lower dose, as this will reduce the possibility of side effects. The following example will show you what can be accomplished.

CASE EXAMPLE

My husband, Len, was discovered to have dangerously high blood pressure and was put onto tenormin tablets (100 mg a day). They had side effects of cold hands and feet and he was always tired. Added to this his asthma was affected, as one of the known contra-indications to tenormin is that it can aggravate bronchial problems. We began an aromatherapy programme with the doctor's sanction and after three months, his tablets were changed to 50 mg per day. This was many years ago, so we were lucky that a doctor allowed the main drug to be reduced, but he explained that people are often given a higher dosage than necessary, to ensure that the problem is definitely under control. He also admitted that not enough doctors reviewed from time to time the intensity of the drug patients were being prescribed. I would like to emphasize that any tablet reduction must be done *only* with the cooperation of your doctor.

The doctor insisted at this stage that Len had his blood pressure taken every day. It was variable for the first few weeks but after three months it had stabilized, so we cut the 50 mg tablets in half, giving 25 mg per day. Again he had to visit the nurse for a daily blood pressure reading until he stabilized. By now he was feeling much better and his side effects were greatly reduced. The final stage of 25 mg every other day was reached a few months later and we were advised by the doctor that this was as far as he was prepared to let it go. It was definitely worth the effort of daily use of essential oils (by inhalation mainly and in the bath, with application on the chest area every night as a supplement). Now, almost 20 years later, his asthma attacks are notably less frequent and occur only in extreme circumstances. With a positive outlook and correct eating, he now only needs his essential oils from time to time for his asthma. I make a tea for him with our own essential oils for high blood pressure (see Useful Addresses). He still takes the reduced dose every other day; even though I feel he no longer needs it, it is not worth taking the risk of cutting it out altogether. I believe in working *with* allopathic medicine and, where drugs are controlled to reduce side effects – and essential oils are also used, for the same purpose (thus making extra drug-taking unnecessary), no permanent damage should be done.

Essential Oils   Juniper, lemon, sweet marjoram, ylang ylang.

Home Treatment   I made a mix of the four oils in a dropper bottle (equal quantities of each). I then added 30 drops of this to 100 ml of our carrier lotion, which mixture he applied to his chest, throat and behind the ears every night and morning; he put six drops of the same essential oils in his bath; I gave him a back massage once a week with three drops of the essential oil mix in a teaspoonful of carrier oil; he cut out milk and dairy products, red meat, pastry and cakes (with regret, and now and again he does indulge in them!) – we started to eat salads every day and plenty of fresh vegetables. I also put six drops of his essential oil mix into a litre of spring water (shaken well each day) and he drank a glass of this every morning.

More and more doctors are willing to try essential oils, particularly to treat secondary symptoms – many nurse aromatherapists write to tell us of successes using essential oils for insomnia or pre-operative stress (see chapter 10), rather than extra drugs which may, of themselves, produce more side effects.

We have talked at length about how to cope in life with 'dis-ease' of mind and body – what about coping with departure from life itself? Much work is done with aromatherapy in hospitals and hospices to help those in terminal care to come to terms with this and to have a better quality of life in those last days. What about help for those who are left behind with their grief? Frankincense, rose otto and sweet marjoram, and also clary and petitgrain, are the best oils to help the bereaved to 'move on' and let go of the past, together with a positive mental attitude that the spirit of the 'lost' loved one is now without pain in the hereafter. Essential oils are also helpful to the nursing staff who work constantly in an atmosphere of grief and despair.

In conclusion, I would highly recommend, if your main problem is severe stress or depression, that you start with one or two professional aromatherapy treatments, if this is viable. If not, then absolute commitment is necessary for your home plan to succeed. Use the fragrant healing powers of essential oils both to soothe and uplift, look at the foods you eat and the thoughts you think – think positive and give God and Nature a chance!

10 *Touch and Essential Oils*

The Right Touch for Massage

Many factors contribute to the achievement of good health and one thing which is not often realized, but which is very important, is that touch also plays a significant part.

To touch means 'physically to come into contact with' and where positive touch takes place with another human being (or favourite pet) it can give pleasure, reassurance, confidence and comfort; no words need be spoken – it is an energy communication. American research this century has proved that people who stroke or touch animals regularly have a better immunity to disease and are less subject to stress than those who do not, and further studies have shown that this applies to babies too.[147] We do not need research to prove to us that the same effects apply to adults; most of us use touch instinctively in one form or another to express delight or compassion and children and adults alike find 'rubbing it better' an almost instant healer, even if, as adults, we mostly rub our own bumps, bruises and headaches!

Even the simplest form of touching is beneficial to the mind – a hand on the arm can sometimes express more than words can say.

Touch does not come easily to some people – a few stiffen or draw back from a hug given as a greeting, or contact during conversation with a 'hand talker'. Perhaps they were not cuddled, stroked or held close during infancy and childhood, or maybe they are afraid to show their feelings; such people, once the door to touch is opened, become happier, healthier and more confident in themselves.

Massage is an extension of touch – caring touch plus time and movement. Its history dates back as far as ancient Egyptian and Indian civilisations – as does plant medicine. Chinese massage is the oldest therapy in the world. Hippocrates, long before the birth of Christ, recorded that a physician should be experienced in 'rubbing' to 'loosen a joint that is too rigid'. We know now that massage 'loosens' the mind too, therefore giving a healing effect to the whole human organism.

Before going deeper into massage movements, there are several points which need consideration, without which the value of any massage could, to some degree, be lost.

Comfort of the Recipient

Let us look first of all at the environment. Make sure that the room is warm and the lighting not too harsh; try to ensure that there are no distractions nearby, or interruptions likely to interfere with your concentration.

Many people use the floor for massage and for shiatsu it is ideal – for aromatherapy it is less so; it is not good for the posture of the giver (or therapist) whose legs and back can become tired very quickly.

Neither is a normal bed an ideal base as a) it is usually the wrong height and b) it yields too easily. A kitchen or dining table is better, provided it is long enough and is made comfortable with a blanket or duvet beneath the top cover. A professional massage couch is the most comfortable for both recipient and giver (after checking the height – see 'Comfort of the Giver' overleaf).

Two towels will be needed, one of which is large enough to cover the whole body from head to toe, or at least from waist to toe. It is much more relaxing for the recipient to have that part of the body not being massaged covered with a towel; moreover, the body temperature falls quickly when lying or sitting still and the towel provides insulation to maintain warmth and comfort. The room temperature comfortable for a therapist may not be warm enough for a recipient, so keep a blanket handy, especially for during massage on the face and scalp.

If carrying out a full body massage, or part massage including the abdomen, check that your recipient has recently visited the toilet.

Pillows add considerably to a person's comfort and are sometimes a necessary support for people of a certain build. Before commencing a back massage, make sure your recipient's feet are relaxed. Sometimes there is a hollow under the ankles – placing a pillow underneath (or a large, soft, rolled towel) will support the feet and help prevent cramp. People with large or heavy chests or an overweight abdomen may find that a pillow placed below or above the area adds considerably to their comfort. When massaging the front of the legs, place a pillow under the head; for the face, chest, arms or abdomen, a pillow under the knees relieves any pressure on the coccyx.

Comfort of the Giver

Make sure you have clean, warm hands and short nails, are comfortably dressed, not wearing high heels or restrictive clothing and have recently visited the toilet to prevent possible interruption. Make sure that you are prepared to give your full attention; having something else on your mind prevents full empathy with the person being massaged.

A professional-type massage couch or table is best – a portable one being the least expensive for home use. The height is of great importance, since your back can suffer if the couch is too high or too low. Ideally, it should be such that, when your hands are relaxed by your side, the top of the massage couch comes roughly to where your fingers join your palm. Many a therapist complaining of backache has found relief simply by adjusting the height of (or changing) his or her massage couch; in a tall person the standard height could initiate backache from bending too low and would create tension in the shoulders of a small person having to reach up.

The stance during massage, if incorrect, can be another cause of backache. Feet should always be apart, their position determined by the part of the body being massaged. When massaging the back and standing on the right hand side of the couch alongside the recipient's right side and facing his or her head – 'north', the right foot should face very slightly 'northwest' with the left foot approximately 18 inches (45cm) behind it facing almost due west, i.e. pointing underneath the couch. The right hip should be about level with the recipient's buttock crease, enabling your arms to reach from there to the shoulders without straining (bending your own back from the base of the spine). A similar stance is beneficial when massaging the front of the leg (using both hands simultaneously); this time the rear foot should be approximately level with the recipient's knee. Check that the toes and top of the thigh can be reached easily (without straining or having to move your feet), simply by a transfer of body weight from the rear to the front foot. This is very important, as your stance should be comfortable and stable enough to prevent you 'walking' in the middle of a movement. See Figure 10.1.

When carrying out massage movements facing across the bed, using alternate hands, the feet should be spaced about 18 inches (45 cm) apart, both pointing under the couch, with the centre of your body level with the half way point of the area to be massaged – this keeps the body balanced.

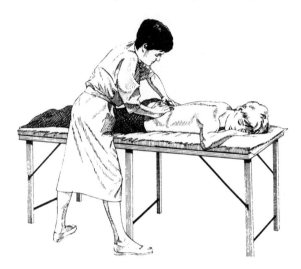

FIGURE 10.1

Aromatherapy Massage Principles

Massage is a therapy in its own right and the use of essential oils simply enhances (doubles) the effect of this already very beneficial therapy. Throughout the ages massage has been given to comfort, relieve pain or relax. Its aims are to increase the circulation of blood and lymphatic fluids in order to increase the release of toxins, to increase or decrease the energy flow of the meridian lines (as in shiatsu), to break down tension in overworked, tired or aching muscles and to tone underworked or weak muscles.

To achieve the first aim, smooth, flowing and continuous movements (effleurage) are imperative; pressure should be applied in the direction of the heart with a relaxed return which maintains full contact with the body.[148] Light, feathery, broken movements will not effect this aim, though they can be excellent in certain circumstances.

The massage used with essential oils (designated as an 'aromatherapy' massage) is principally traditional massage (without percussion, except in particular cases where it may be needed) enhanced by a small amount of shiatsu, lymph drainage, neuro muscular and connective tissue massage. Each of the latter techniques is a complete and specialized massage treatment in its own right and to carry out such a treatment in full it would be necessary to attend a course on the specific subject.

Shiatsu massage works on the principle of energy flow and is dependent on the mood and character of the person being massaged. Those who practise both shiatsu and traditional massage often ask about the importance of pressure towards the heart, as in shiatsu, working on energy lines can involve pressure in the opposite direction also. The answer has to be that many shiatsu movements cannot be mixed at random with aromatherapy massage, which selects only a few of those which work on certain pressure points, *after* the blood circulation has been increased. Shiatsu movements are also usually performed at a much slower rate.

Lymph drainage massage is carried out on the superficial tissues, following the direction of the lymphatic circulation towards groups of lymph nodes (located in special areas throughout the body which filter off bacteria and toxins transported there). Movements like these are carried out in aromatherapy to help improve the lymph flow and accelerate the release of these toxins.

Neuro muscular massage involves stroking or friction movements following the nerve pathways and entails working on specific areas of tissue which feel different from normal, to improve both the nerve and the blood circulation. It is very similar to connective tissue massage, which employs pulling and stretching of the various soft tissues of the body.

'The superficial tissue of the skin is richly endowed with nerve endings and changes in this connective tissue, e.g. inflammation, congestion, precedes many chronic diseases.'[149]

Empathy

In any form of massage the depth of caring of the giver and the trust and belief of the recipient play an important part in the end result of the treatment. The therapist should be giving his or her whole attention to the client who is sharing the experience. This does not mean taking on their problems or their emotional state. All too often I hear therapists saying they are 'drained' after treating a needy client. There is all the difference in the world between sympathy and empathy. Sympathy is feeling sorry for someone (and can be destructive); empathy imparts the feeling that someone cares enough to help the person to help him/herself. A good therapist will listen, support and encourage, but should not take the client's problems on board.

What's In a Hand?

Everything! Many books say one should have soft hands for massage. It is certainly a bonus if they are, but it is far, far more important to have *relaxed* hands. Over the years I have met with long, thin hands which massage beautifully and short plump hands which cannot – yet *all* are capable of touching and stroking another human being in a friendly, caring or loving way – it just takes time for some people to learn how to relax and use their hands to the best advantage. Occasionally I find that even people qualified in massage carry out an upward effleurage movement with pressure on their fingers. (This is where soft, plump fingers would at least have some advantage over long, bony ones!) Such tension and pressure from the wrong part of the hand (effleurage) is uncomfortable – and sad if this is the client's first experience of massage.

Imagine a lovely oak parquet floor and two people of identical weight walking on it. One is wearing stiletto heels; the other, flat heels. You do not need me to tell you the damage done to the floor by the person whose body weight is concentrated on only a tiny area. In massage, the fingers are the stiletto heels and the palms the flat heeled shoes!

Imagine now that your forearm is the handle of a floor mop and your hand the mop head. A mop head is floppy – an efficient, gentle cleanser, moving wherever the person holding the handle directs it; it is not sharp, hard or tense – hands should be as relaxed as this! I said 'the person holding the handle' to illustrate that the handle itself does not do the 'directing'. In massage, the muscles of the arms should not be tense – the body weight (leaning on the hands) should direct the arms. Now stand in front of a mirror, bend your elbows and relax your hands. You will notice that your fingers are not touching each other. Concentrate on the feeling when you bring your fingers together. Can you feel the muscles in your hands and forearms tightening? Relax them again – and see how much better you feel.

Before starting to massage check to see if you can maintain this relaxation whilst moving along part of someone's body. The back is a good place to try this. Put a little oil on your hands, rubbing them *briefly* together only long enough to cover them completely and to warm the oil before spreading it on the back. Stand comfortably and correctly, bend your elbows, relax your hands, then gently lower your forearms until your fingers (keep them floppy!), then your wrists, are touching the lower back. Your fingers should slightly face one another – not point directly towards the head of your client; this could make your muscles tense. Check that your fingers are still relaxed and separate; then forget they are even there, focusing all your attention on your palms. Let your body weight (from the shoulders) give the necessary pressure to the palms as you direct them up the back to the shoulders. Keeping your fingers relaxed and floppy and still in full contact with the body, move your hands across the shoulders ('cuddling' them) (see Figures 10.2 and 10.3), and continue the journey back to the lower spine, gently relaxing the pressure as you go by, releasing your body weight; your palms and relaxed fingers should cuddle the *sides* of the body all the way down, with full palm and (relaxed) finger contact.

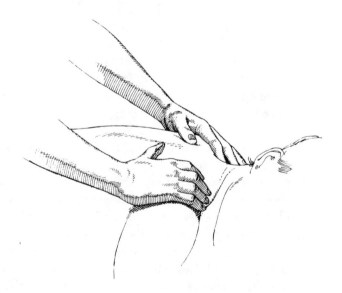

FIGURE 10.2

When you have mastered your stance and pressure (using your body weight) and can give a completely smooth and relaxed movement on the back, you can tackle anything!

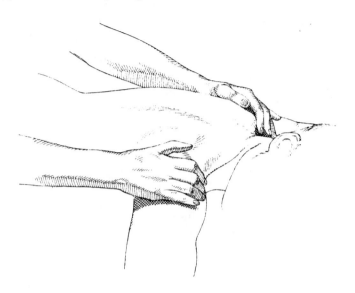

FIGURE 10.3

Prime Factors of Massage

The all-important considerations when giving massage (particularly full body) are contact, continuity, pressure, rhythm and speed. Contact and pressure have been covered above, so let us look at continuity. Once contact has been made, your hands should remain on that section of the body until you have finished massaging it. If essential, you can lift off one hand, but never both. The reason for this is that each time you place your hands on the body, the nerve endings of the recipient can sense the 'landing' and there is a slight break in the relaxation.

Many people love watching ice skating or ballroom dancing – the smooth rhythm resulting from long practice is relaxing and harmonious. The movements of those who are just learning the art would be jerky and uneven and would not give the same pleasure to the onlooker. To be enjoyed to the full (and to receive maximum benefit), there should be a smooth rhythm in massage movements too.

The speed of an individual massage movement can be varied to suit the effect you are wishing to achieve, be it to stimulate or relax. However, the overall speed of the complete treatment should neither be taken at a gallop nor at a snail's pace. It is impossible to give an 'average' speed – one needs to watch a massage being done to assess this. Should the recipient need to relax, slow overall speed is preferable; the speed should not exceed approximately seven inches (18cm) per second so that the desired effects can be obtained,[150] otherwise you risk putting your client into a state of agitation rather than relaxation.

Main Massage Techniques

Effleurage

Effleurage is made up of two movements - deep stroking, a smooth, firm and fairly slow movement towards the heart, followed by a light, relaxed return, as learned in 'What's in a Hand?' above.

Effleurage plays a leading role in any massage, being the most soothing, and although there are many variations which can be effected on all parts of the body, the principle remains the same. Effleurage in some form should be given both at the beginning and end of each group of movements completed on any one area, and is often executed also in between the other types of movements employed.

Petrissage or Kneading

This is a more energetic movement, involving moving the hands or fingers closer together to squeeze gently parts of a muscle or muscle group. This can only be done where there is enough flesh to pick up easily. It involves both hands working together, using the palm and the whole length of the fingers, or the thumb and fingers, depending on the size of the muscle being massaged. It should always be preceded by effleurage, to relax and warm the area first and should be gentle but firm, without any break in contact. Tense muscles respond well to kneading and the movements promote the blood circulation locally. It is difficult to describe and is best learned in a teaching situation. See Figures 10.4 and 10.5.

Petrissage (or kneading) greatly increases the blood circulation and removal of waste products and is very effective around the shoulders, where most of our muscle tension is held.

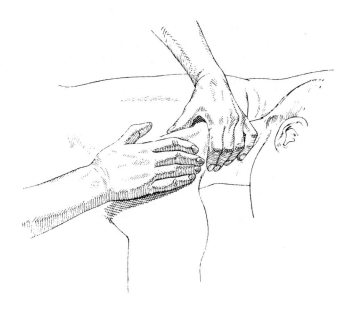

FIGURE 10.4

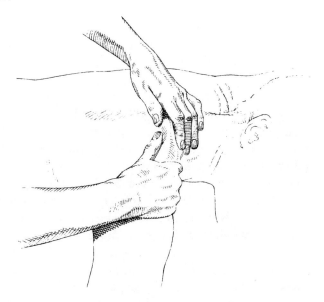

FIGURE 10.5

Frictions

Frictions are usually carried out with the soft cushion of the thumb, though they can also be done with the fingers and, on large areas, with the heel of the hand. The part of the hand in contact carries out deep circular movements over the needy area (without losing contact) and may glide along a specific path while circling. Frictions help to break down fibrous knots and tension nodules, increasing the peripheral circulation substantially. See Figure 10.6.

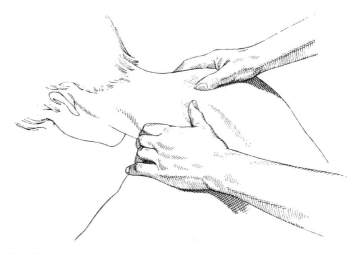

FIGURE 10.6

Aromatherapy massage concentrates mainly on these three types of massage movements and only in special circumstances employs percussion. 'Percussion' describes its performance exactly; the ulnar border of the hands (while open or cupped) or sideways fists are 'banged' in rapid (alternate) succession onto the body, like drumsticks on a drum. It is said to help break down fatty tissue, but I feel it would need to be carried out for at least an hour a day to be effective in this respect!

Effleurage is the fundamental skill of all massage, which is why I have gone into the details of its basic movement. Once this is mastered, other effleurage strokes can be learnt easily. My other books, *Practical Aromatherapy* and *Aromatherapy for Common Ailments*, each give details of massage movements for the layperson and there are several good books specifically on massage (see Further Reading). A would-be aromatherapist will cover the more difficult aspects of an aromatherapy massage when he or she takes an aromatherapy course.

Nevertheless, after giving some of the contra-indications against massage, I will detail both a neck and shoulder massage which can be done at home on another person (very effective for the relief of stress and its resulting muscle tension and headaches) and a self-applied shoulder massage (excellent for nightly self-treatment, and demonstrated on the video I made with my daughter Penny).

Possible Contra-Indications to Massage

There are occasions when it is inappropriate to carry out an aromatherapy massage, which may occasionally be contra-indicated, or need special care – the following is a guide on some points of which to be aware.

1. Infectious or contagious diseases (no massage at all)
2. Running a temperature (no massage at all)
3. Recent fractures and large areas of scar tissue (no massage over that area – wait two to three months. Gentle application of essential oils in a carrier is a great aid to scar healing, minimizing the scar and keeping it supple)
4. Varicose veins (very gentle massage, using only upward effleurage)
5. Cancer and serious heart conditions (no full body or back massage – unless with permission from the doctor; shoulders, arms, hands, face and feet can be massaged)
6. Broken skin, boils, cuts (if small, simply cover with clear, fine sticking plaster)
7. Recent inoculations (wait at least 24 hours – longer if problematic)
8. Recent alcohol intake (massage and essential oils together can heighten the effect of the alcohol, possibly causing dizziness or a 'floating' feeling)
9. Straight after a heavy meal (the body is concentrating on digestion and a full body massage or abdomen massage could cause nausea; other individual areas may be massaged)
10. If very hungry (full body massage could cause fainting)
11. Immediately after sport, a hot bath or sauna (the body is exhaling and cannot absorb the essential oils – wait ½–1 hour)

12. The first two days of menstruation (the blood loss could be acceler-ated; local massage to soothe pains is helpful. Individual areas may be massaged)

13. If on strong (and varied) medication (no full massage without doctor's permission; individual areas may be massaged).

Pregnancy is not a contra-indication to massage (though often quoted as such) – indeed it is most beneficial during the whole nine-month period. Naturally, care has to be taken as the baby grows and the massage adapted accordingly; for example back massage is more comfortable lying in the 'flapping fish' position (one arm behind the back, the other in front, resting on a soft pillow and level with the head).

If you know you or your client is pregnant chapter 6 will help you to select the oils which are best to use during this important period.

Giving a Neck and Shoulder Massage

Let the client sit on a comfortable stool or upright chair (not too high-backed) and with a pillow if choosing to sit facing the chair back for added comfort. (Special massage chairs are available for back and shoulder massage.)

Add three to four drops of essential oil to a teaspoonful of carrier oil (or use a little from a previously mixed bottle). Place a little of the blended oils into your hand, briefly rubbing both hands together before applying the oil into the neck and shoulders.

1. Placing hands gently at the base of the shoulder blades (facing slightly inwards) effleurage up and around the shoulders and upper back (with whole hands), repeating several times to warm up the area (see Figure 10.7). Finish with fingers on shoulders and keep them there.

2. Reach down your thumbs as far as they will go comfortably. Circle firmly using thumb friction movements in the hollow on either side of the spine, moving right up to the neck. Without lifting off your fingers, return to base and repeat (see Figure 10.6 on page 206).

3. Move round to the side of the chair to face one shoulder square-on, and place your hands gently onto the shoulder (see Figure 10.8). Move each hand in turn up to the neck (one behind the other, rhyth-mically) in smooth effleurage movements. (Because the hands follow

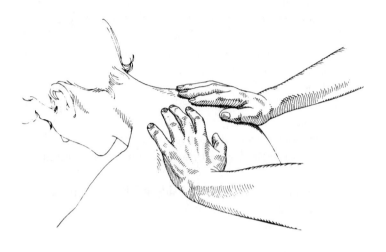

FIGURE 10.7

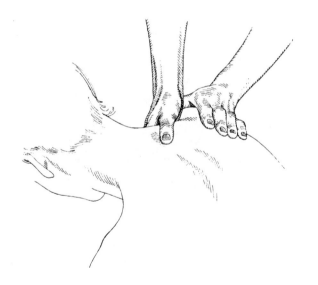

FIGURE 10.8

one another each may be lifted off at the neck as soon as – not before!
– the other has commenced its stroke.)

4. Feel on top and behind the shoulder for nodules or tense tissue, doing
   firm thumb circles on these. (Keep the other hand still, in contact
   with the body.) If the shoulder muscle is very tense alternate the
   circles with movement 3 to give moments of relief.

5. Placing the hand nearest the front of your partner gently on his/her
   forehead (for balance), take the other hand up the back of the neck,
   'squeezing' firmly as you do so and relaxing down to the base of the
   neck before repeating three or four times (see Figure 10.9).

6. Return to the back of the chair and repeat the first effleurage movement.

7. Walk round to the other side of the chair to repeat movements 3, 4
   and 5 on the other shoulder.

8. Repeat movement 1.

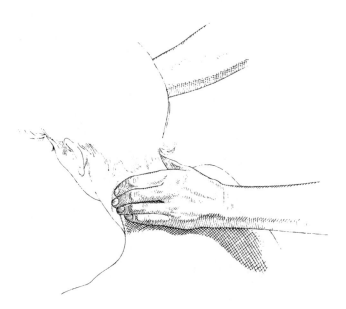

FIGURE 10.9

Self-Applied Neck and Shoulder Massage

This wonderfully relaxing 'massage' is one you can give yourself every night before getting into bed, to ensure a relaxed physical state, resulting in a deeper and therefore more beneficial sleep. If you have difficulty sleeping, take a 10-minute bath first with essential oils, or inhale them either from a tissue or a vaporizer for at least half an hour before carrying out the routine below and going straight to bed.

Use a non-greasy lotion base for your essential oils unless you want to spend a long time on yourself (or prefer a carrier oil). Mix three to four drops of essential oil into a teaspoonful of your chosen base and put half into the palm of your hand (or use from a previously mixed bottle). Rub your palms briefly together and apply to each shoulder.

1. Stroke your left shoulder firmly in circular movements with the whole of your relaxed right hand (your hand should 'drape' over your shoulder), starting on the edge of your shoulder and moving gradually up to your neck.
2. Push your fingers into the tight muscles on and behind your shoulder – you will soon find those nodules which hurt – and make small firm circles over the the painful areas. See Figure 10.10.

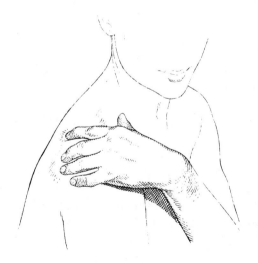

FIGURE 10.10

3. Repeat no. 1.
4. Take your hand up the side of your neck, making circular movements with your fingers and finish behind the ear.
5. Repeat no. 1.
6. Repeat the whole sequence with the left hand on the right shoulder; use the other half of the mixture the following night.

Touch and Aromatherapy in Hospital

An Introduction

Friends, relatives and other people in hospital or a hospice derive great benefit from being touched – especially with essential oils.

The best known and accepted form of touching another human being is by a handshake. Apart from being a friendly gesture, it tells us a little about a person and is an ideal starting point for massage for those neither familiar with, nor certain about, this art. It is a good way to introduce essential oils to someone who does not as yet know much about either the oils or massage. When we lecture at hospitals, I usually suggest to nurses the following procedure – which can be done by anyone.

Carry with you a small bottle of carrier oil containing a 2 per cent mixture of two or three relaxing essential oils and just before entering the room, apply a little to the palms of your hands.

Suggested recipes, in 20 ml carrier oil:

2 drops juniper	or	3 drops geranium
2 drops marjoram		2 drops sweet orange
3 drops lavender		2 drops lavender

(The first recipe is also helpful for rheumatism or arthritis.)

When you say 'Hello Mary – how are you feeling today?' take her hand as in a handshake (without the 'shake') placing your left hand on top of hers (see Figures 10.11 and 10.12). All of us have many technical skills, but forget how much good we can do, or how much pleasure we can give, by just a few minutes of touching and holding someone's hand. After a few minutes Mary will probably make some comment regarding the aroma, at which time you can let her smell your hand. If you get a positive response you can begin to move over her hand and even up her lower arm in an effleurage movement (see Figure 10.13). This small sequence makes a talking point and also leaves Mary with a pleasantly relaxed feeling and a lovely aroma – which must be beneficial. If your friend does not know about your interest in essential oils, you would explain as you took her hand.

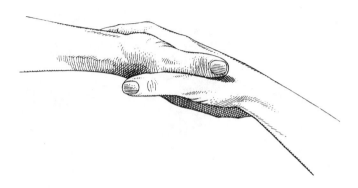

FIGURE 10.11

Hospital patients who have difficulty sleeping can be helped with touch and essential oils. This time take an oil mixture to your evening visit containing sleep-inducing essential oils and use the same hand approach with massage – on both hands.

Suggested recipes, in 20 ml of carrier oil (macerated lime blossom oil could be helpful here as the carrier – see chapter 8):

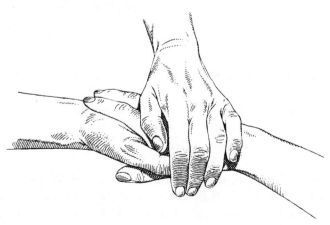

FIGURE 10.12

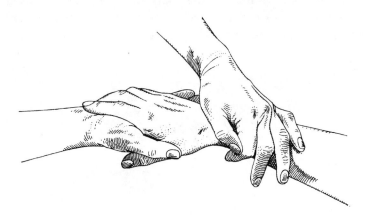

FIGURE 10.13

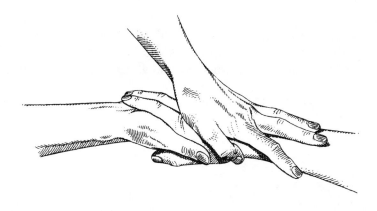

FIGURE 10.14: Finish by stroking firmly right down to the fingertips, making a 'sandwich'.

3 drops lavender   or   4 drops lavender
2 drops ylang ylang   2 drops Roman chamomile
2 drops sandalwood

It would be helpful to apply gently some of the same oil on the forehead also and behind the ears. Alternatively, put a little on your friend's hands so that he/she can apply it all over the face and neck (including behind the ears – a very good spot for penetration).

Foot massage is a natural progression from hand massage and is one of the most relaxing and healthful 'treatments' one can give, though not always the easiest to give successfully. It is extremely important to hold the foot firmly all the time, giving firm movements; many people do not like their feet to be touched only because they think it is going to tickle; a light grasp or light movements can also feel quite unpleasant.

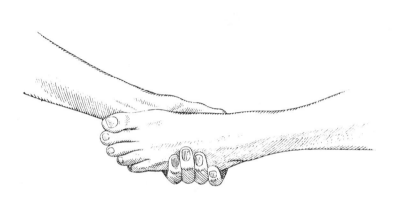

FIGURE 10.15

Holding the foot in a 'sandwich' is the best way to begin (see Figures 10.15 and 10.16), as it involves the whole foot and, to get a perfect result, the right hand should finish, after effleurage of the lower leg, on top of the patient's left foot (vice-versa on the right foot), both hands squeezing together as they move towards the toes (see Figures 10.17 and 10.18). Bring the lower hand to the top of the foot, while turning the upper hand (as shown in Figure 10.19) and recommence massage.

Where people are visiting a relative or friend who is about to have (or has had) a serious operation, or who is terminally ill, I often suggest they ask the nurse if she would like to put some relaxing essential oils into a vaporizer. Vaporizers for use in hospitals should be electric, as these are safer for children and old people (nursing staff would not be allowed to use a night-light vaporizer). If a vaporizer is not available, put a few drops of the selected essential oils into a tissue, to be inhaled regularly (it can be lodged in your friend's nightgown or shirt or under the pillowslip if he/she is lying down). Many nurses have told me not only how beneficial this has been to all concerned, but that people often ask permission to use essential oils on their relatives in hospital where it is not being done by the nurse.

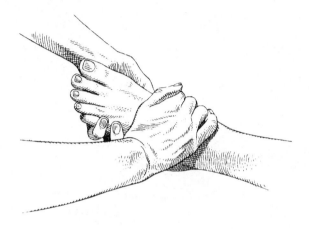

FIGURE 10.16

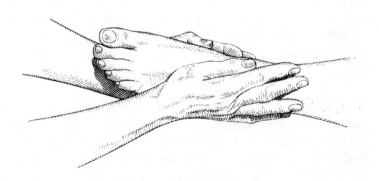

FIGURE 10.17

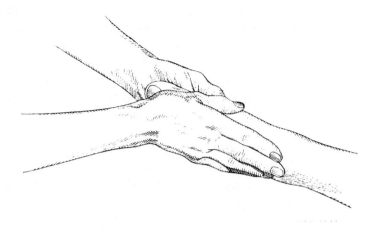

FIGURE 10.18

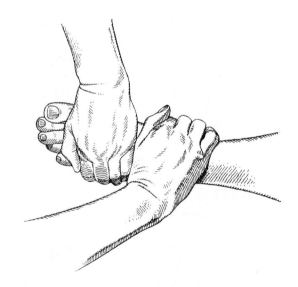

FIGURE 10.19

CASE EXAMPLE

Thomas aged three, had to have an operation for an undescended testicle. His mother, an aromatherapist, wanting him to have a good sleep the night before his operation, put one drop each of sandalwood and lavender in his bath and massaged him also with these oils. Within four minutes he had dropped off to sleep. Before he went down for his operation the next morning she massaged the solar plexus reflex area of Thomas's foot with the same mix, to keep him calm.

The nurse in charge told Thomas's mother that children on the ward often suffer from insomnia and she was so impressed by Thomas's reactions to aromatherapy, she obtained permission from the consultant to purchase electric ceramic vaporizers and essential oils to use on the ward.

Various Uses in Hospital

Len and I lecture at hospitals all over the country, including those where aromatherapy is not yet used; a high level of interest is shown by nurses (and some doctors) and a significant proportion of students of aromatherapy comes from the nursing profession. In those hospitals where it is used, we are told enthusiastically about the wonderful results; many nurses, after qualifying, have persuaded their consultants and doctors to allow essential oils to be used on the wards instead of some secondary drugs.

Aromatherapy is used generally in hospitals to help with problems such as insomnia, whether it be due to stress on account of the unfamiliar surroundings or due to the side effect of a particular drug being administered; it is used to relieve muscle cramps, help mothers-to-be on the labour ward – the list is endless! It is even used to de-stress visitors and the nurses themselves.

In one Scottish hospital a study has been carried out on patients in the rheumatology ward. As a result, a lotion to help arthritis is now officially administered on the ward and an approved research project is being set up in the same hospital.[151]

Several intensive care units, many hospices and cancer care wards now use essential oils – aromatherapy does not 'cure' the patients there, but it makes a tremendous difference to the quality of life enjoyed by those suffering from terminal illnesses.

One nurse, concerned about the more clinical approach to nursing nowadays, is delighted (as I am) that aromatherapy allows nurses to touch patients and develop the caring side of their profession. She finds that after massage with essential oils, patients in intensive care under sedation and bombarded by lights and strange noises, have a reduced anxiety level, become less confused and are more aware of their surroundings. It also reduces any side effects of digestive upsets such as constipation.

I wish that all hospitals had consultants interested in complementary help for their patients – that time will come, I am sure, judging by the rapid growth in hospitals of aromatherapy purely since the beginning of the 1990s!

Caution

I would, however, like to offer some advice to nurses who are not qualified in aromatherapy, and do not have an aromatherapist nurse, or visiting aromatherapist working in the hospital. Please do not attempt to try any essential oil on a patient without knowing exactly what that particular oil is capable of in those exact circumstances. Essential oils are powerful in their concentrated state and have already been misused in hospitals by nurses with insufficient knowledge about the oils themselves and how they may be used (see chapter 6). We are all keen to see these wonderful oils accepted in general practice and hospitals throughout the country, but negative experiences will retard this progress.

One of the associations (IFA) has a special 'Aromatherapy-In-Care' group working in hospitals in the UK; another (ISPA) has people working in hospitals in the UK and in Uganda (where all the drugs donated have passed their 'sell-by date'!) In these latter hospitals, some of the aromatherapists work non-stop, treating people who have walked (or been carried) 8 or 12 miles because they have heard about the 'new' treatment.

The Royal College of Nursing has set up its own Special Interest Group to look further into the introduction of complementary therapies into hospitals. Not only that, but the General Medical Council have given doctors the authorization to delegate specialist functions, treatment or procedures to complementary therapists, provided the doctors retain ultimate responsibility for the management of the patient and are satisfied as to the competence of the therapist. This will lead eventually to a more holistic health approach all round, to the benefit of all concerned.

In 1997, at the suggestion of HRH the Prince of Wales, a discussion document (Integrated Healthcare) was published by The Foundation for Integrated Medicine, to consider the current position of orthodox, complementary and alternative medicine in the United Kingdom. Its aim is to investigate the possibility of the public having access to a wider range of effective and safe forms of treatment and aromatherapy is one of the therapies where impressive developments have been made in terms of self-regulatory structures, improved standards of training and greater public recognition.

The discussion document identifies the call for 'a common body of knowledge and skills which all health-care practitioners need'. This echoes the view the Author has had for several years now that there should be a basic curriculum which all would-be complementary practitioners should complete before studying the discipline or disciplines of their choice – this would ensure uniformity in the basic skills required by all complementary practitioners in order to practise their therapy or therapies efficiently and knowledgeably.

11 *Women's and Children's Problems*

Menstrual Problems

Attaining womanhood is a complicated business, bringing the onset of the often problematic blood loss each month. Some girls are lucky and sail easily into womanhood with only the inconvenience of the loss itself, but many suffer fear or embarrassment, pain, irregularity or menorrhagia (extra heavy flow). Those unlucky enough to suffer from PMS as well spend almost a third of each year living in semi-discomfort with a nuisance factor. I know I have painted a rather bleak picture, but what many women have to put up with every month of their lives is what I hear most about in my job!

I can remember in my late teens spending almost two days each month in agony; tablets were not freely given then, nor had I discovered essential oils. I lay alternately curled up with a hot water bottle or pushing my feet hard against the bottom rail of the bed; at school I suffered in lessons and was unable to take anything in.

Nowadays (if you do not want to take painkillers) essential oils can provide the perfect answer. The most effective oils for women's problems are, unfortunately, the more expensive ones – particularly true melissa and rose otto. Roman chamomile and clary are next on the price scale and a mix of two or three of these four (where indicated) can give excellent results.

Using aromatherapy necessitates active participation on your part. To reduce pain or blood flow and for regularizing your period, essential oils should be applied in a carrier every morning and evening on your tummy and the small of your back for seven days before your period is expected to start (10 if you are sometimes early). You can also put six to eight drops in your bath. Do not expect perfect results the first month – by the second or third you will notice the difference. Neither should you be dismayed if, after three months, there is not much improvement; people react differently to different essential oils in just the same ways as they do with allopathic tablets. Simply look at the therapeutic reference again (in chapter 14) and try a different mix of oils.

Some essential oils have the ability to encourage the body to increase its production of oestrogen; among these are aniseed, fennel, niaouli, sage and clary sage.[152]

PMS

(Sometimes referred to as PMT or pre-menstrual tension)

Pre-menstrual syndrome (syndrome = a set of symptoms) is a fairly common problem, directly connected with stress, which is itself a recent 'malady' (increasing as the emancipation of women has brought more responsibilities at work or the stress of bringing up a family on their own). Such a lifestyle has made many women more susceptible to PMS and the symptoms are many and varied.

PMS is a combination of mental and physical symptoms which affect women anything from two days to two weeks before a period and usually at the same time of the cycle each month. The list of symptoms can be enormous, and could be any of the following: bloating of the abdomen (connected with the congestion usually responsible for painful or over-heavy periods) depression, facial spots, fatigue, fluid retention, food cravings , insomnia, inability to control emotions, irritability, severe headache (even migraine), tender breasts and weight gain. Fortunately, it is rare for all symptoms to manifest themselves in a single individual!

It is thought that the increase in the number of PMS sufferers may be due partly to diet changes over the last century. Nowadays, we consume great quantities of sugar, alcohol, tea, coffee, dairy products and animal fats; excessive intake of products containing caffeine can increase anxiety, stress and even insomnia.

A high intake of sugar and sweets does not help the PMS sufferer (do you have an urge for chocolate just before a period?) An increase in appetite and/or sugar craving, perhaps a week prior to a period, may contribute to weight gain and fluid retention.

We consume enough salt naturally without adding more to food in cooking or at the table (how many automatically reach for the salt pot before even tasting the food?) Following a healthy diet, including vegetables that are natural diuretics, such as cucumber, cabbage and fennel will be of great benefit (when you cook fennel do not throw away the water – drink it!). Plenty of salad and fresh fruit will help your digestion to work efficiently and prevent unnecessary build-up of the acids which can be formed to the detriment of your well-being.

Another important fact to take into consideration is exercise. If you do not care for time-consuming exercises a simple solution is to jog on the spot for one minute every morning when you get up (see chapter 9). It is surprising how effective and stimulating this can be, and it keeps your circulation flowing well. Other exercises good for PMS sufferers are walking, swimming, aerobics and yoga. Yoga is not only a physical exercise – it helps reduce the all-powerful mental stress level!

The level of minerals present in the body is important, especially that of magnesium, which in PMS sufferers is often found to be low. The conditions contributing to PMS, which magnesium helps to reduce, are menstrual cramps, blood sugar levels and mental depression. Nuts – cashews, almonds, brazils, peanuts (see chapter 8 on carrier oils) – provide magnesium naturally.

The emotional part of PMS is the worst. One little utterance from another person and the sufferer is in a flood of tears or so angry she could burst a blood vessel! In this area essential oils are of tremendous benefit because of their almost instantaneous effects when inhaled. At this stage of PMS, anything up to seven days before a period, try an essential oil mix of Roman chamomile, lavender and clary – the salvation of a friend of mine. She shakes a few drops onto a tissue and inhales deeply – the effect is calming and the aroma wonderful! You may prefer a different aroma (many oils can balance the emotions) though I would suggest you incorporate Roman chamomile or clary into your choice of oils. Roman chamomile is known for its calming qualities, clary is uplifting and lavender creates an aromatic balance, as well as being therapeutic. For a really exotic and effective blend one could use rose otto! Rose otto is well known for balancing problems connected with the reproductive system.[153]

Endometriosis

This name is given to a condition where 'clumps' of tissue from the lining of the uterus (the endometrium) appear in parts of the body other than the uterus such as the ovaries (the most common site), fallopian tubes or even the bladder. The condition can be the cause of excessive blood flow at menstruation, painful periods, painful intercourse and sometimes infertility.

Treatment is not easy and sometimes surgery may be advised. Aromatherapy has been found to be helpful; one of our staff and one of our teachers avoided surgery by using essential oils. It is a distressing condition and both felt that the oils helped to lift their spirits, which is a good beginning to any aid to health. The hospital staff were surprised at the reduction of 'lumps and bumps' on one of them after she had followed the aromatherapy treatment for three or four months. Each had her own mix of oils, putting into a dropper bottle one of the recipes given below. Both followed the same routine: six drops in the bath, and 15 drops in 30ml of carrier oil or lotion, a little of which was rubbed into the small of the back and abdomen every day. Each had a foot reflex cream containing their oils, with which they massaged each foot for five minutes daily on the solar plexus area, followed by the reproductive and excretory areas.

2 ml each	3 ml each
cypress	geranium
geranium	clary
sage	rose otto
sweet thyme	

Vaginitis

This is inflammation and irritation of the vaginal tract together with a discharge, sometimes caused by leaving a tampon in too long, taking the pill or other steroid drugs, or occasionally due to infection through a trichomonas microbe (from a type of venereal disease), when the discharge is a greenish-yellow. The most frequent cause is fungal infection with candida (a yeast) when the discharge is whitish (see thrush below). Sitz baths with two drops each of tea tree essential oil (for the infection), lavender and sandalwood (for the inflammation and irritation respectively) will be found to be effective, as is application twice daily of the same essential oils in a carrier oil or lotion.

Thrush

Thrush is caused by a yeast-like fungus called *Candida albicans*, a normal occupant of the mucous membrane of the mouth, the intestines and the vagina. When the body's defences are low this yeast becomes more active and takes the form of white spots in the mouth or a discharge from the vagina. Tea tree essential oil (being anti-fungal as well as antiseptic) has been found to be an effective cure for this in the early stages; it can be put directly onto a tampon (it has not been found to cause any skin irritation – despite its strength as an antiseptic), which should then be inserted for a minimum of two hours or overnight. Sitz baths using the oils for vaginitis are also recommended. If the immune system is low, essential oils should be used to boost this and strengthen it against infection.

Menopause

Cessation of activity by the ovaries usually occurs around the age of 50, though it can begin several years earlier. Many women sail through it with no trouble, although some experience problems such as excessive blood flow and hot flushes (including the occasional embarrassing situation). Normally the periods gradually become less frequent (with decreased flow), or cease suddenly as mine did. Symptoms presented by the less fortunate are due to the adjustment in the production level of oestrogen, which their particular system cannot cope with.

Emotional stability is often affected, with hours of depression and a drop in self-confidence. Physically, hot flushes (including sweating during the night) and dryness of the vaginal tract seem to cause the most discomfort. Hot flushes are caused when the reflexes controlling the blood flow are temporarily out of balance, causing a sudden surge of blood resulting in an increase in temperature. Hormone (oestrogen) Replacement Therapy (HRT) is believed to be the answer to all these problems and in the majority of cases, it halts the physical symptoms, including helping to prevent the onset of osteoporosis (when the bones become weaker and more brittle), and thinning of the skin.

Dr Ellen Grant, who has carried out much research on oestrogen tablets, is concerned that continued HRT could encourage the formation of cancer cells.[154] My advice is always (unless an illness is acute) to try essential oils first – there are quite a few hormone balancing oils. You have nothing to lose and with careful, controlled use there are no side effects.

Hot Flushes

These are perhaps the worst of the physical afflictions, arriving without warning, but you can help them to go more quickly using essential oils. Prepare a bottle of peppermint water by adding four drops of peppermint essential oil to a litre of spring water. Shake well twice a day for two days, after which it will be ready for use. Fill a small bottle from your big one, and keep in your handbag together with a few circles of cotton wool. The moment you feel the onset (or straight afterwards) drink nearly all your peppermint water, leaving enough to dampen a cotton wool circle with which to pat your face (the most embarrassing area affected by the hot flush). A small handbag spray filled with peppermint water is ideal to cool you down quickly (make sure you keep your eyes shut). As a preventive measure, try to have a regular back massage (professional or by a friend or partner) using two drops of each of cypress, clary and lemon, with one drop of peppermint in 20 ml of carrier oil. Use the same essential oils in a lotion for regular self-application on the small of the back and abdomen. (One to two drops of lemon oil can replace one peppermint drop in the water formula if liked.)

Conception

The monthly shedding of the uterus lining indicates that a girl is now fully developed and capable of bearing a child. The majority of women prefer the pill to other forms of contraception – it is without doubt the most efficacious, but unfortunately completely changes the hormonal balance of the body (and offers no protection from venereal disease or AIDS).

At the age of about 35 I was put on the pill to regularize my periods (which arrived when the fancy took them – from 2½ to 5 weeks apart). That inconvenience was immediately eased, but a few months later I began to have the side effect of migraines a few days before each period. These were thought by my doctor not to be a result of taking the pill, but of the period itself and my age! To alleviate them I took migraine tablets for two days, which became a habit I accepted as normal. After 10 or 12 years I went to the doctor (a new one) for my first cervical smear test and she was horrified to find me still taking the pill, the prolonged taking of which she told me could possibly bring about cancer. She did not renew the prescription and after three or four months my migraines disappeared.

It is important to wait at least three to four months after coming off the pill, before attempting to conceive,[155] as it is not fully known how the pill affects the egg production or the eggs themselves. The chemicals from the pill are retained in the body for a while and may affect the baby (research has identified dyslexia as being a possible result), so it is worth using a physical method of contraception (such as a diaphragm or condoms) for three or four months. Also, after a number of years of being on the pill the reproductive system becomes so accustomed to the abnormal routine of perpetually preventing the release of an egg that it can sometimes be difficult to conceive.

Knowing this, couples should not then worry regarding failure to conceive at first, otherwise a vicious circle may begin, as worry causes stress, making it even less likely that conception will occur.

Before I entered the world of aromatherapy I noticed time and again that some couples, having established that neither was physically incapable and having tried for years to have their own baby, adopted one. Very soon afterwards the wife became pregnant, a possible explanation being that now they had their baby, love-making was a more relaxed affair.

It is not so easy to adopt babies nowadays, and stress increases when there is no conception. It makes the muscles of the body tense and circulation is impeded; in the case of infertility, the muscles in the reproductive area are tense, perhaps preventing a full flow of sperm, reducing vaginal secretion and even giving the egg a slower journey down the fallopian tube so that it is not in the right place at the right time.

Using essential oils just before love-making will not only relax these muscles (along with those of your whole body), but give the emotions a chance to relax and uplift too. Even if a physical reason may be hindering conception, it is well worth using essential oils; their use can only enhance your love-making and relieve any guilty feelings which may be felt by either partner (see next section).

Infertility

In these days of stressful living, more and more couples seem to be having difficulty starting a family. One of the problems is that some want to have a nice home, a car (or maybe two) and all modern conveniences first, the wife has probably been taking the pill to ensure that no babies come before they are financially established. This alters Nature's course of events and has an effect on fertility when the pill is discontinued (see previous section).

Amenorrhoea (lack of periods) is a natural hindrance to fertility, stress sometimes being responsibility for a temporary cessation. Irregular periods can also hinder conception if the condition is really acute and not just a matter of being six to 10 days late.

There are all sorts of physical problems which can cause infertility; low sperm count, lack of eggs in the ovaries, narrow or blocked fallopian tubes, to mention but a few. Some of these may need medical help but can also be helped with aromatherapy.

Sprinkled on a tissue and inhaled, essential oils have a profound effect on all kinds of mental and physical problems, and though there has not been much research as yet on the use of essential oils for infertility many aromatherapists, including myself, have had some success in this field.

CASE EXAMPLE

At a party, some time ago, I met Paula, who had just gone through the trauma of divorce after three years of marriage (no children). Her periods (which had not begun until she was 16 and were never very regular) had become scanty and few and far between. She was about to remarry and was anxious to start a family as soon as possible.

Our hostess at the party had told her how aromatherapy had helped her own painful periods and had suggested she ask if I could help her with her menstrual cycle.

Aromatherapy needs the total co-operation of the person concerned and a lot of hard work, as treatment has to be carried out daily; Paula was more than willing to comply with this.

The essential oils I chose were German chamomile, true melissa and rose otto, undiluted for use in the bath every other night. I gave her the same recipe diluted in a white lotion base to apply every night to her tummy and lower back.

After about six weeks of treatment Paula had a fairly normal period (which she may have had in the normal course of events anyway), but when the next one came about eight weeks later, followed by another after a six week gap, she was happy to continue with the treatment. It took about a year for her period to come every four or five weeks and just before her second anniversary she and her husband had a beautiful baby girl. (They now have a little boy too.)

CASE EXAMPLE

A couple had been longing and trying for a baby for two or three years and had undergone many tests. They had become very stressed (particularly during Lucy's fertile days), which was making their love-making a strain instead of a pleasure, with Lucy not even wanting to take part. They visited one of our trained aromatherapists (with a natural gift for understanding personal problem areas), who put into a small bottle essential oils of clary and ylang ylang, which are not only relaxing but said to counter frigidity. Lucy loved the aroma blended for her (which is in itself a very important part of the treatment) and was happy to use six to eight drops in her nightly bath. The same oils were put into a carrier oil to be applied by each partner onto the other at the beginning of love-making, starting with the shoulders and whole back. (Women often take longer to become aroused than men, so the man should massage his partner's back first, then she his. He can then massage her abdomen before she does his, after which it will be a mutual and personal progression.)

This helped both Lucy and her husband to approach each other in a more caring way without making the desire for a baby the only reason for their love-making. Lucy was amazed at how much she enjoyed her massage and how it actually made her want to be an equal participant, making the whole sexual experience happier, more loving and more relaxed. I do not have the outcome of this story yet, as it is only a few months since treatment began but I am sure there will be a baby in that family before very long.

Essential Oil Choice

Trying to select a blend of essential oils pleasing to both partners is interesting, as what may smell lovely on one person may not give off the same aroma on another. We all have a slightly different level of skin acidity (which affects any perfume or essential oil aroma applied), so I cannot give you 'set' recipes – I can only suggest oils that most people would find relaxing and arousing. It is important that the final aroma is one you love, so the proportion of each oil in a mix must be a personal choice; it can only be arrived at by trial and error, using only one or two drops at a time. (Make a note of what you are adding each time!)

For a woman: clary, sandalwood and ylang ylang make a lovely synergistic mix.

For a man: bergamot, geranium and black pepper blend well together.

For both: to give more confidence and positivity try bergamot, rosemary and neroli (or petitgrain distilled over flowers - if you can find a good supplier).

When you have discovered your recipe, make up a little bottle of concentrated essential oils for the bath and add about four drops of this to a teaspoonful of vegetable carrier in an eggcup for massage.

Once you have found a blend which 'turns you on' use it also in a vaporizer (see chapter 7). Put it in the bedroom at least an hour before bedtime to give the room a chance to fill with the aroma.

For ways of impregnating bed linen with essential oils, see chapter 12.

Pregnancy

I well remember the feeling when I was told I was pregnant – a wonderful moment, followed by slight apprehension about what was to follow (my mother lived 200 miles away). I was lucky, working till the end of the seventh month and suffering no morning sickness – only backache and very bad varicose veins (in the family anyway!) Nowadays there are essential oils which can help these characteristics of pregnancy (and more!) – I do not want to call them 'symptoms' – pregnancy is not an illness!

There is a lot of talk nowadays about which oils to avoid during the first few months (or the whole) of pregnancy. This information is of the most relevance to couples where the woman has been taking the pill for a long time or where a miscarriage has already been experienced – in other words, those who are *aware* of trying to conceive. The risk is very slight in any case, **when using essential oils in a normal and correct fashion.** It is only if women overdose themselves in order to force a miscarriage in the early months that certain oils may (or may not!) actually give the wanted result. When a woman tries to bring on an abortion by using essential oils in hugely excessive doses (i.e. 20–50 drops two or three times every day *internally*) she could do more harm to herself – the baby could survive unharmed![156] However, in the normal course of events, the essential oils would not be used in such huge quantities and therefore would not be hazardous to either mother or child. Unfortunately, as information has already appeared in several books and magazines, mostly without this full explanation, those presentations will no doubt stick in people's minds, frightening some unnecessarily.

My overriding concern is that because of the excessive publicity (without full facts), those wishing they were not already pregnant will try all the oils mentioned in the hope that they will abort. This is not guaranteed to happen – they could simply make themselves seriously ill.

A paradox of this situation is that women do not necessarily know for at least six weeks after conception that they are pregnant, yet this is the very time when so-called 'toxic' essential oils would be more effective (i.e. hazardous).

Be aware of the potential hazards of some essential oils, use them carefully and, at the same time, keep the published exaggerations in perspective.

In *Aromatherapy for Common Ailments* I had to mention every single oil that may have even a *slightly* detrimental effect[157] because the book was written for the American market, and the recorded attempts at abortion through use of essential oils come from the USA.

Not all the oils suggested to be avoided are emmenagogic (producing menstruation) – some are neurotoxic (having a strong effect on the nervous system) or hepatotoxic (having a strong effect on the liver), and I think that if information is to be given regarding hazardous oils, the full story should be told – 'a little learning is a dangerous thing!' These special oils are not going to over-stimulate the reproductive and nervous systems, or the liver, unless carelessly, thoughtlessly or purposefully used with intent to cause harm. Any hazard pertaining to these oils applies all through pregnancy up to the last four to six weeks, when some, sensibly used, can be helpful. Some otherwise harmless essential oils are best not used until after the first five months (see Table 4, Powerful Oils, in chapter 6) in case they are used incorrectly from the baby's point of view.

Now, having got that off my chest, let us look on the positive side – how essential oils can help some of the problems of those people who are happy to be pregnant.

The First 7½ Months

During the first three months, medication of any kind should be avoided where possible, emphasis being placed on diet, exercise and sleep pattern. Food intake should be adjusted to include plenty of natural, fresh, unrefined foods, wholemeal bread and lot of fresh vegetables and fruit. Cigarettes and alcohol are best left alone, as they can adversely affect a pregnancy (far more easily than can essential oils!).

Morning Sickness
The first inconvenience to be noticed early in pregnancy may be nausea, not only in the morning but sometimes as a result of inhaling certain aromas occurring in everyday life. Pregnant women have a heightened sense of smell and this can contribute to the feeling of sickness, especially during cooking, or being in the company of a smoker![158] A low fat, sensible diet is a big help for morning sickness.

Essential oils of petitgrain and mandarin (or sweet orange), when used in a vaporizer or on a tissue, can be a great help towards preventing or eliminating nausea. If a handkerchief or cotton wool ball with four drops of petitgrain and two of mandarin (with one drop of sandalwood to hold the aroma and also contribute to the effect) is attached to a pillow at night, the smell will linger until morning, thus lessening the possibility of morning sickness. As an alternative, it is a good idea to put these same oils with water into a vaporizer and leave in the bedroom overnight. If you take a bath first thing in the morning, add four to six drops in total of mandarin or sweet orange and petitgrain.

A well-known cure for both nausea and heartburn (see below) is peppermint (only one drop is needed) and many proprietary brands of indigestion tablets include essential oil of peppermint in their composition. If using peppermint, be sure to use a complete oil; a folded one may be too strong for a pregnant woman (see peppermint in chapter 4). Add a maximum of two drops of peppermint to the other oils of your choice.

True melissa is a traditional French remedy for morning sickness, used as above or in a tea (see chapter 7), or make an infusion with the leaves if you have the herb in your garden (much less expensive!)

Heartburn

As the baby grows, pressure on the stomach may cause occasional indigestion in the form of heartburn. Sandalwood (in particular), petitgrain, sweet and bitter orange, mandarin and lemon are all excellent aids to the relief of heartburn.[158] The simplest method of use is inhalation. Put two or three drops of sandalwood together with two or three drops of one of the other oils onto a tissue and take deep breaths. Another effective method is to make a tea (chapter 7). Alternatively, use the oils in a carrier (quantities given in chapter 7) and massage firmly for several minutes in a clockwise direction over the painful area, using the palm and heel of the hand.

Stretch Marks

How I wish essential oils had been available in this country when I had my children! Unsightly stretch marks can now be prevented with twice-daily use of essential oils in a carrier oil. Since I came into aromatherapy, every person who has applied my stretch mark oil daily has survived with a smooth, unmarked skin.

Important considerations to bear in mind, in order to have 100 per cent success:

1. The carrier oil base should include calendula or hypericum (St John's Wort) oils (or both) for full skin benefit.
2. The oil mixture should be applied every morning and every night from the end of the fourth month (or from when you feel the baby move) until six or seven weeks after the birth.
3. As the baby grows, so the area covered should be increased, including eventually the breasts, upper thighs and sides of the body. The skin above the breasts often becomes stretched by their weight, so include the upper chest early on.

Any regenerative essential oils are good here, such as frankincense, myrrh or lavender (not so effective on its own). It is a good idea to include an oil

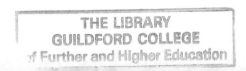

which is a tonic to the skin, such as lemon or mandarin, and black pepper, which is a tonic to the muscles.

Back Pain

This is something from which I suffered myself and is easily alleviated with the use of essential oils. To ease general spinal stress throughout the latter half of pregnancy, take a relaxing bath for 10–15 minutes and/or apply a mix of essential oils (two drops each of Roman chamomile, sweet marjoram and lavender) in 10 ml/two teaspoons of carrier to the painful area, asking your partner to do it for you if it is difficult for you to reach. The same oils can relieve pain in the groin area due to the strain on ligaments towards the end of your pregnancy.

Constipation

It is imperative, as the baby grows, to be sure and keep your bowels regular and easy. How I wish someone had told me this little gem! If you have back pain as well, choose essential oils which are helpful for both conditions (see suggested recipe below), thus killing two birds with one stone. Eat plenty of fresh fruits and vegetables, wholemeal bread and fibre-rich cereals to maintain a healthy evacuation routine.

2 drops black pepper
2 drops sweet marjoram
2 drops Roman chamomile
    in the bath or massage in 10 ml/2 teaspoons carrier

Emotional Imbalance

Many conflicting emotions can occur during pregnancy (both confusing and upsetting for the mother), such as volatility of mood and slower brain reactions. State of mind can have an effect on the foetus and, by caring for the total self while pregnant, the growing baby can be nurtured effectively in the womb, ensuring it will be calm and healthy.

Geranium and mandarin are good 'balancers' of mood and together make a most effective aroma used by inhalation (see morning sickness), or in the bath (four to six drops in total). Rose otto and clary are effective here too.

Insomnia

As the baby develops, the mother may experience difficulty dropping off to sleep. Inhalation using two or three drops each of sandalwood and ylang ylang are most useful as an aid to relaxation. These oils can be put in the bedroom in a vaporizer, inhaled from a tissue or used in a warm bath an hour before going to bed.

Varicose Veins

Whether or not you are prone to these, you should keep watch each month to see if any are commencing and take immediate action if they do. Most advice given to pregnant women in the latter months includes resting in the afternoon (if possible). For those with a tendency to have varicose veins, may I say from experience that rather than rest the whole afternoon, it is more beneficial to lie on the floor, raising your legs onto an easy chair, for five minutes in every half hour. This prevents the vein walls from overstretching due to long periods of standing with extra body weight on them and is easier to accomplish than lying down all afternoon if you already have children.

As an extra help, apply essential oils in a carrier oil or lotion (in an upward direction) just before you get out of bed in the morning and after each, or every alternate rest period with your legs in the raised position. As a preventive measure, use your mix twice a day in the manner just described. Unless you prefer to use my mix (Care for Visible Veins), lemon, cypress, neroli, niaouli or clary are helpful – see recipe below. Sandalwood and peppermint (maximum two drops) in the mixture will soothe any irritation and can be used for haemorrhoids too, if you are unlucky enough to have these after the birth.

50 ml carrier oil or lotion
5 drops cypress
5 drops lemon
3 drops niaouli
2 drops peppermint
1 drop sandalwood

The Last Six Weeks

Preparation for Labour

Rose otto and fennel are excellent for strengthening the womb and the Braxton Hicks' contractions. Sage and fennel are not harmful at this stage, if employed in the dilution recommended. One of the best methods of use is in tea, one cupful two or three times a day for the last month. You can now add three to four drops of clove bud or rose otto to your stretch mark oil to help the uterus gain strength and tone.

Labour

The big moment has arrived! Hopefully you have already attended pre-natal exercise classes and perhaps your partner has decided to be present at the birth – a marvellous experience for him, guaranteed not only to bring the two of you closer together, but also to give him a deeper bond with his child. Giving birth is a wonderful experience and should be looked upon not as painful but as hard work, because that's what it is! If you can manage to do without anything which makes your senses muzzy, please do – essential oils are a good substitute for gas and air.[158] Put a few drops of clary on a tissue or ball of cotton wool to hold in your palm all through labour. While you have longer than 15 minutes between contractions, lie on your side and ask your partner or whoever is with you to massage your tummy gently in a clockwise direction (and/or the soles of your feet) with previously prepared oil in a little bottle.

Suggested recipes in 20 ml carrier oil:

2 drops each: clary, rose otto, ylang ylang
2 drops each: Roman chamomile, mandarin, sandalwood

At the same time, just before you think a contraction is due, breathe in deeply two or three times from your clary tissue. After each contraction breathe in the essential oil gently and rhythmically until the next one starts. As the time between each contraction reduces, and you feel you can manage without gas and air, begin to use your tissue or cotton wool ball as though it were the gas and air machine. Some people put the cotton wool into the switched-off machine because it 'feels better'.

New Mother

Birthwounds

If you have been torn, damaged with forceps or cut during the birth, a sitz bath of cypress (to help stem the blood flow) and lavender (to hasten the healing) will give results so quickly the nurses will be quite impressed![158]

Milk Flow Difficulties

For those who have insufficient milk and want to be able to breastfeed, apply one drop of fennel in 10 ml/2 teaspoons carrier lotion three times a day to your breasts immediately after feeding (not on the nipples), to ensure complete penetration before the next feed.

Mastitis

To help prevent mastitis, always first offer the baby the breast you used last at the previous feed. If you have too much milk, hand-express the surplus after feeding to prevent congestion. Roman chamomile, clary sage and peppermint in a carrier oil will help anyone who is unfortunate enough to develop mastitis. A compress of the same oils is very soothing and quickly helps to return the breast to normal (see chapter 7). Always use baby strength dilution (i.e. 5 drops in 50 ml) on the breasts if breast-feeding.

Weaning

When you are ready to wean your baby over to cow's milk and baby foods, cut out one feed a day first, then two; the last one to go should be the bedtime feed. Oils of cypress, lavender and peppermint in a lotion on your breasts will help reduce the flow of milk if you have a problem (always apply just after feeding, twice a day).

Babies

Note: Rather than continually using he/she or her/him, the baby is a boy throughout.

Essential oils should never be given to a small baby internally. However, a massage or application with suitable essential oils in very low dilutions (5 drops in 50 ml) is not only beneficial to many baby problems (and completely without hazard) but ensures a happy baby. To use in the bath mix 5 drops essential oil into 1 teaspoon of honey and gradually add water up to 50 ml. Use 1 teaspoonful of this in a baby bath or 2 teaspoons if bathing the baby in a normal bath. Babies only need very weak mixtures to be effective.

Keeping Babies Calm and Relaxed

Babies soon learn to associate a smell with love, warmth and comfort, so it is worth while putting one drop of sweet smelling oil such as mandarin or geranium on a tissue near the baby whilst feeding.[159] This works if children are fretful in the night; in this case put the same aroma on a tissue beside them, or put two drops on their night clothes; it will calm them down, helping them to get back to sleep.

Babysitting Difficulties

If you give the babysitter a similar tissue to the one above, he/she will have a much easier job!

Wind

If you are blessed with a greedy and therefore windy baby, massage your breasts (not nipples) with two drops of mandarin or bitter orange, one drop of Roman chamomile and one drop of peppermint (to keep well below the skin sensitivity limit) in 30 ml of carrier lotion one hour before feeding the baby. Also, and if you are not breastfeeding, use the lotion to massage the baby's back and tummy. Wind is often the cause of colic in babies, so preventive treatment is a good idea.

Colic

A baby prone to frequent wind for long periods of time is said to have colic. Prevention is better than cure so try to ensure your baby is neither taking in a lot of air with his feed, nor is too hungry, causing him to rush his feed. Use the Roman chamomile mix mentioned above and burp baby frequently while feeding. It is a good idea to put on a compress after feeding, winding and changing.

Put one drop of Roman chamomile into a screw top jam jar with an inch of water and shake well. Add about ¼ inch hot water, stir well and soak the compress in it. Place on baby's tummy, covering with a square of cling film. Keep in place with the nappy and wrap a warm scarf all around.

Wakefulness

The amount of sleep a baby needs varies from one to another. So long as your baby is happy, do not worry about him not sleeping or eating as much as your friend's baby. If he is dry, well-fed, yet crying a lot (not stopping when you pick him up), it is best to seek advice. To encourage sleep, an hour before putting him to bed put a vaporizer in the bedroom (where he cannot reach it) with a few drops of lavender or/and Roman chamomile or petitgrain, or keep a tissue with these oils under the pillowcase covered by the sheet, removing the tissue just before laying baby down.[160]

Nappy Rash

Even happy babies will cry if their nappy is wet or if they are left regularly in a wet state. A mass of little red spots indicates that nappy rash has developed. In place of baby oil apply the following mix to soothe the irritation and clear the skin. Blend two teaspoonfuls of calendula oil slowly into 40 ml (about eight teaspoonfuls) of carrier lotion. Add two drops of sandalwood or rose otto, two drops of lavender and, if you have it, one drop of German chamomile – this last is excellent for the skin. Use this mix as a preventive measure at every nappy change; a baby's waste matter is quite acid and easily 'burns' the delicate skin. Alternatively, use my Soothing Balm.

Teething

One of the most painful experiences for a baby, apart from colic, is the production of teeth. For years, clove extract has been used by dentists (and still is) to deaden toothache. It is an oil which should not be used neat on the skin as it may be an irritant. However, in the extremely weak mixtures advocated for babies there is no hazard whatsoever. If you are not an aromatherapist, ask one to mix this for you. Put one drop of clove bud oil into an eggcupful of carrier oil (approximately 20 ml), stirring well with your finger. Run your finger (moistened with the mixture) round baby's gums several times a day to soothe the pain. The mixture can also be applied externally on the area concerned.

Insomnia

If for any reason, baby gets into a habit of waking up, or if he is not a good sleeper, use one drop each of lavender and Roman chamomile in 20 ml of carrier oil to massage his back before putting him to bed. Put the same oils in a vaporizer – well out of reach – and light it (or switch it on) about ½ hour before bedtime. Alternatively, put four drops each of the same essential oils onto a tissue and place between the sheets for ½ hour before bedtime (when it should be removed).

Emotional Problems

If you are breastfeeding, how *you* feel affects your baby. If you are cross or depressed, he will cry more; it not only affects your milk flow but your emotional feelings will come over in your physical and verbal contact (this, by the way, also affects bottle-fed babies).

Many new mothers suffer from post-natal depression, some so deeply that they do not want anything to do with the baby. If you feel 'a little low' at *any* time, it is worth nipping it in the bud, by inhaling essential oils of true melissa and/or rose otto. Should you not have one of these, lemon, clary and sandalwood together are a reasonable substitute. Put your oils onto a tissue, into a vaporizer, into a bath – anything which will make you feel better. This is very important, as depression, if allowed to take hold, can weaken the immune system. New mothers are not 100 per cent stable healthwise for about three to five months after giving birth and when the immune system is low, vaginal thrush may more easily develop, presenting another possible problem to be coped with and cleared up.

Essential oils are extremely helpful both in strengthening the immune system and getting rid of thrush (see therapeutic references in chapter 14) but better by far, when you need your health for looking after baby (perhaps other children too), is to begin using essential oils immediately you feel emotionally unstable.

Children

For most children's ailments the same choice of essential oils can be used as for an adult with the same problems; they will be found most effective for earache, toothache (see 'teething' above), coughs and colds, tantrums, burns, cuts and bruises, etc. Do not use any oil which may cause skin irritation or sensitivity, and up to the age of 13, halve the number of drops of essential oil (to go in the bath or a carrier) that would be used for an adult.

Childhood Conditions

When little ones need calming or have been exposed to infections use essential oils (they are excellent preventives).

Two drops of each oil from any one condition listed below, can be used in a third of a bathful of water per child aged three and over. One drop of each in a quarter of a bathful of water per child under three years old. For massage or application use 8 drops of essential oils in 50 ml of carrier oil or carrier lotion.

Calming	Lavender and Chamomile
Chicken Pox	Lemon and Lavender
Colds and Coughs	Tea tree and Eucalyptus
Colic	Orange and Chamomile
Insomnia	Sandalwood and Lavender
Measles	Eucalyptus and Lavender

12 *Oils at Work in the Home*

General Health Safeguards

All essential oils are antiseptic to some degree, many also possessing powerful bactericidal properties. Recent research at the Scottish Agricultural College has revealed the effectiveness of savory and tarragon essential oils to counteract the development of several different bacteria, including those significant to public health.[161] Previous microbiological studies have proved most essential oils to be at least as powerful as carbolic acid (phenol) – some many times stronger.[162] Peppermint oil, equal to carbolic acid in preventing the spread of bacteria, is a well-known ingredient in mints and other confectionery, including throat tablets. Compared with carbolic acid lavender oil has a factor of two – meaning it is twice as powerful. Moving up into the 'heavy brigade' we have clove oil (used by dentists) with a factor of eight.[163] Obviously effective, clove is used to curry meat in hot countries. Other essential oils have factors of 12–15, including fennel, *phenolic* thyme and tea tree. The latter two are very powerful, with aromas to match (the addition of citrus oils, geranium or lavender helps them to smell much sweeter).

Some powerfully antiseptic and bactericidal oils need to be used with care and should not be available over the counter where there is no aromatherapist to advise. Because of this, I have chosen oils for use in the home which are without hazard, still powerful and the most reasonable cost-wise.

Your own health should be your first concern. Germs usually multiply in a body which is run down, stressed or abused in some way, lowering its natural resistance to infection or illness. Do not encourage these germs by ignoring simple techniques which would prevent them from spreading;

keeping the house germ-free when it (or you) is exposed to germs, is quite simple and visitors will love the aroma your home emanates. Two drops each of sweet thyme, lemon and pine (the latter is an excellent air anti-septic) in a vaporizer or on a tissue for personal use will keep germs at bay.

You can spray or vaporize relaxing oils in the lounge and bedrooms, fresh-smelling ones in the bathroom, and spicy, herby ones in the dining room and kitchen. All rooms can then attack invading germs and keep their occupants healthy.

In these days of widespread use of harmful pesticides and fertilizers, and advice telling us we shouldn't eat this and we shouldn't drink that (because of cholesterol, sugar, additives or colouring etc.), anybody who takes their health too seriously could starve! Bacteria abound and contam-ination is everywhere. The air we breathe, the water we drink, the food we eat – none is sterile, and all are a potential source of illness!

Before you give up and despair let me assure you that we cannot live without friendly bacteria – it is only the *un*friendly ones to which I refer. In any case, if we lived in a sterile environment we would have no oppor-tunity to build up immunity and would succumb to every little germ.

We have at our fingertips some powerful natural allies which are very user friendly – namely, essential oils! To use essential oils in the home makes good sense, and it also makes good scents!

The Kitchen

Unseen dangers lurk here – why not make your kitchen hygienic, safe and aromatic! Essential oils are a real pleasure to use, with the bonus of leaving the air smelling delightfully fresh and clean.

The least expensive essential oils come into their own here. Lemon, bitter orange, grapefruit, cedarwood, petitgrain, tea tree – choose any two or three to give the aroma you prefer. I mix 2 ml each of lemon and grape-fruit and 1 ml of petitgrain in a little dropper bottle, using three to four drops from this in a basin of water. I wipe my kitchen surfaces with a cloth rinsed in this, occasionally adding a couple of drops of tea tree or cedar-wood (if I fancy a woody aroma). A single essential oil has a dramatic hygienic effect, but a mixture of two or three not only makes a synergistic and more effective mix, but can be blended to create the aroma of your choice.

Dishcloth

A likely source of germs is the most used item in the kitchen – the dishcloth. Dishcloths are notorious hoarders of germs and ideally a clean dishcloth should be used every day. It should be boiled regularly to kill all germs and rinsed in water containing four to five drops of your essential oil mix.

Dishes

If you want to use essential oils in your dishwasher, they are best added to the rinse aid, shaking well before use (you would need 3 ml for a 250 ml bottle). Human dishwashers derive an added benefit; the essential oils in washing-up water evaporate upwards, creating a pleasant aroma and killing bacteria at the same time!

Chopping Boards

Wooden chopping boards are great germ hoarders, used as they are for chopping and cutting raw meat, cooked meats, bread, vegetables, etc. The porous surface soaks up bacteria, providing a very comfortable home for them! You may possibly clean your chopping board thoroughly under a running tap and scrub it (if you use a wooden one) – but how often is it sterilized? Put four to five drops of your essential oil mix into a quarter of a cup of water and pour it over your board after cleaning it, leaving it to drain or wiping it with your aromatic dish cloth. Even a plastic board should be sterilized – *and* the chopping knives!

Fridge

The fridge lining can absorb odours from the foods inside. Keep it fresh by cleaning it (and your whole fridge) with water containing the essential oil mix, finishing with the aromatic cloth. Always check the fridge is cool enough to render bacteria inert.

Floor

When it comes to washing floors, tea tree is a must, adding oils such as petitgrain or cedarwood if you want to enhance the aroma. Six drops of tea tree plus three drops of one of the others is adequate for a bucket of water and be sure to treat your floorcloth with essential oils, as the dishcloth above!

Ironing

To make your ironing smell fresh, although lavender is traditional, try adding two drops of lemon and/or grapefruit oil to a spray bottle of water, shake it well, then spray each item lightly before ironing. Do not be tempted to put essential oils in the water reservoir of a steam iron as it may eventually craze due to undissolved globules of essential oil.

General

To give a nice aroma to the kitchen and as a gentle antiseptic, use your essential oil mix, plus 2 drops pine, in a vaporizer, or fill a spray bottle with water plus six to eight drops of your favourite oil or oils, shaking well before use.

Personal Hygiene

Do you wash your hands before you begin to prepare a meal? What about the children's hands when they help collect the ingredients and roll out the pastry? It is imperative that hands should be washed before handling food, particularly raw meat (after which they and the utensils should be re-washed), otherwise there is a danger of cross contamination. Fingernails, especially long ones, are a favourite place for germs to collect.

Cooking

In the Middle Ages, before ice machines and fridges were thought of, meat was kept from putrefying by the use of traditional herbs, which not only helped to preserve the meat and protect the stomach from infection, but also added a distinctive flavour, to help to disguise any 'off' note the meat may have had – so common in those days (hence mint with mutton, sage with pork, etc.)

The same herbs are still used in modern cooking, but to add flavour rather than to hide any unpleasant taste. Essential oils are easy to use and, unlike fresh herbs, can be stored for long periods of time without losing any of their potency. They are, however, much more concentrated and need to be used very sparingly (see the end of this chapter).

We can protect ourselves (and our stomachs) from attack by unfriendly bacteria, e.g. salmonella and listeria, by cooking or reheating food thoroughly. (It is best to avoid eating too many foods which need reheating.) Make sure you know how to use the microwave oven correctly. The cook should also take precautions to protect the family when suffering from a sore throat, stomach upset, cut or skin abrasion. You obviously cannot stop cooking for your family just because you have a sore throat, but essential oils can be used against anything which may be 'going the rounds' at school, at work, or at home. By gargling (see chapter 7), spraying the room just prior to cooking and observing basic hygiene rules, the cook can reduce any risk of passing on infection. Before cooking, wipe the worktops with water containing your essential oils.

Burns

How many times have you burnt your hand or forearm when using the oven, iron or electric hob? Lavender is a wonderful gift to those who burn themselves. First of all, run your hand under the cold water tap; this takes away the heat and stops the flesh from 'cooking'. One drop of neat lavender on the burn after cooling with water diminishes the pain and healing starts immediately. A bad burn, not serious enough to require medical attention, should then be treated by diluting 10 drops of lavender in half an eggcupful of carrier oil or lotion, applying this mix several times a day.

Living Room/Lounge

Carpets

Carpets, particularly those in heavy traffic areas, quickly collect germs from outdoor shoes and pets and could be a danger to babies at the crawling stage. How many people remove outdoor shoes before entering the house? In one or two families I know this is still the rule, though it may be to keep the floors clean and the carpets from being worn, rather than any thought of reducing bacteria (we do it to protect our wooden floor)! The kitchen mix of essential oils in half a pint of water and sprayed onto the carpet after hoovering will keep your carpets germ free.

Atmosphere

Use relaxing or uplifting essential oils in a vaporizer, spray, or on the radiator (see chapter 7), to set the mood for a party or create a soothing atmosphere after a traumatic day.

Open Fire
In the winter, you may like to try putting two or three drops of essential oil on each log stacked at the side of the fireplace for your evening's supply. The aroma of base note oils lasts longer than that from top notes because of the slower evaporation rate (larger molecules; remember chapter 3?) A dropper bottle containing 10 drops of sandalwood and 20 each of cinnamon and nutmeg gives a good spicy aroma. If the heat is fierce, the oils will evaporate quickly, much of the aroma going up the chimney (depending on your fire) and you may not find it a very efficient method.

Bedroom

Health and Happiness
Essential oils are needed most in the bedroom either to help health problems or to de-stress personal relationships (see chapter 11).

Bedlinen
Essential oils can be put into the washing machine (for bedlinen or clothes), though I have not had much success this way. If you wish to try it, mix the essential oils in fabric softener, using this in the softener compartment of your machine so that the oils go into the rinsing water. Do not put neat essential oils into the compartment as they can affect certain types of plastic (usually the brittle kinds).

You could also take some dried flowers and lay them onto a large handkerchief. Sprinkle with essential oils, gather the corners and edges together, securing with a piece of thin ribbon or an elastic band. Shake well and put your pot-pourri in between the sheets in the linen cupboard.

For an occasional treat, put the pot-pourri hanky, or a drop or two of essential oils, on the inside top edge of the duvet cover or sheet when you change the bed linen. Your choice of oils depends on what function you want them to fulfil, so refer to the therapeutic charts in chapter 14.

Drawers and Wardrobes
Using essential oils here is for pleasure rather than for health, though there could be a slight health benefit, depending on the oil used. For drawers, put one drop of essential oil in the centre of each quarter of a drawer liner or on small strips of paper and leave for an hour in the closed

drawer before putting in your clothes. A pot-pourri handkerchief (as above) can be put in between the clothes instead, if preferred.

For wardrobes put the essential oils onto a small piece of cotton wool or kitchen roll, pushing it onto the metal hook of every third or fourth hanger. Use only distilled or expressed oils – and not lemongrass, as this, and resins and absolutes, could stain your clothes.

Bathroom

Hygiene
You can use the kitchen essential oil mix here, especially for the toilet; three to four drops of nice-smelling oils can be put into the bowl after cleaning e.g. pine, lemon.

Baths, Jacuzzis, and Hydrotherapy Baths
The section on water as a carrier in chapter 7 tells you in detail how to use essential oils here.

Holidays

Packing
Put one or two drops of your favourite essential oils (or mix) onto a couple of paper tissues (or on the lining of the suitcase – do not use absolutes or resins on this or deep coloured essential oils such as lemongrass) and leave inside the suitcase for a day before packing. The tissues can be left in if you want a lingering aroma.

Pre-Travel Stress
For many people, the process of 'going on holiday' can give a multitude of stresses – what clothes you should take, whether or not you will have a stomach problem, will mother be well enough before you leave, and so on. Much pre-holiday stress can be diminished by carrying a tissue around with you sprinkled with any relaxing oil or oils from the reference charts in chapter 14.

Travel Sickness
Pack a little first aid kit of essential oils: peppermint, ginger and caraway are three to help settle your stomach before and during a long journey.

Peppermint works well on its own, but if you want a synergistic mix, put 20 drops of peppermint and 10 each of the other two into a dropper bottle. Before you leave, put three drops from the mix into a teaspoon of carrier oil or lotion and rub some onto your chest, stomach and behind your ears. During the journey, put a few drops from your bottle onto a tissue and inhale from time to time.

Hotel Rooms

It is a good idea to take a small spray bottle with you on holiday. We do a lot of travelling and occasionally have been given a room which smells either musty or of cigarette smoke. I carry a dropper bottle containing a mixture of geranium, nutmeg, ginger and clary. I use about 10 drops of this mix in a tiny spray bottle with water immediately, and by the time we have had a meal, the room has either no smell, or an aromatic one.

Suggested recipe:

10 drops geranium
4 drops nutmeg
3 drops ginger
3 drops clary

The number of drops can be adjusted to give an aroma acceptable to each individual.

I have a friend who, whenever she arrives in her bedroom (however luxurious the hotel), turns back the bed linen and sprays the mattress with a solution of red thyme (cedarwood may be used also) to kill any bacteria or bugs which may be there! It sounds absurd, but she and her husband were once bitten by bed bugs in a reputable hotel – once bitten, twice shy!

Stomach Upsets

A dropper bottle containing fifteen drops each of peppermint, ginger and sweet fennel, with five drops of sandalwood makes an excellent mix for an upset stomach. Use this neat for inhalation and put three to four drops in a litre bottle of water, shaking well each time before use. When travelling to a Mediterranean country such as Egypt or Morocco, the litre of water is a must – we are never without one, using it as a preventive with great success. If you suffer from travel sickness too, use these oils for both problems. It is quicker for stomach upsets if you make a tea (chapter 7) and drink a cup every couple of hours; however, if this is not possible, inhale the oils from a tissue at regular intervals and add three drops to a teaspoon of carrier oil or lotion (if you have remembered to pack some!), massaging it onto your stomach (in a clockwise direction) and the small of your back at frequent intervals.

Sunbathing

The ultimate aim of many holidaymakers is to get as brown (or as red!) as possible, as quickly as possible. Redness can be prevented in one of two ways; a few weeks before leaving home visit a suntanning centre, to build up some resistance to ultraviolet rays; if this is not possible, try to be patient and introduce your body *gradually* to the penetrating and relentless rays of the sun. However good a sun protection product is, it is foolish to expose yourself for more than two half hour sessions on the first day (one hour sessions if you have a skin that browns fairly easily). Gradually increase the daily exposure time by half an hour each time (one hour for the hardy). Going red and sore benefits no-one, and you will probably peel. Sunbathing is not a good idea these days anyway as it can lead to skin cancer if overdone. Tops of feet, thighs, shoulders, necks (especially below the throat) and noses are the most vulnerable areas and should be well covered with an efficient sun product at regular intervals (my sun milk has made many people happy over the years, especially those who cannot tan easily or who normally break out in a rash). If you do overdo it, be prepared with the recipe below, applying it at regular intervals until you no longer feel sore. The same mix can be used before going into the sun, but whatever you use, do not be tempted to stay there too long at the beginning of the holiday!

Suggested recipe in 100 ml white lotion:

8 drops German chamomile (4 drops if you do not like the aroma)
8 drops lavender
5 drops sandalwood
4 drops peppermint

Miscellaneous Methods of Use

Paper Money

How often have you opened your wallet or purse and twitched your nose distastefully? Apart from the smell (or because of it!) paper money is most unhygienic. Choose your favourite essential oil and put one or two drops onto a narrow strip of paper. Place this in your wallet or purse – and the shop assistants will have a pleasant surprise when they take your germ-free, aromatic money!

Books
There are several reasons why using essential oils in a book is a good idea, apart from sheer pleasure. Most of us pick up a book when we need to relax, and relaxation is enhanced by the inhalation of certain essential oils – simply choose the one which gives you the most pleasure. If you like to read before going to sleep, oils like lavender and ylang ylang would be ideal. When studying, and wishing to keep your mind active and awake, peppermint and rosemary would be an excellent choice.

If you use a bookmark put one drop of essential oil on the lower end; if not, put one drop of oil near the beginning, the middle and the end of your book – close it and leave for a while to permeate the pages (not lemongrass, absolutes or resins – these will stain the pages).

Birthday Cards and Letters
To give an extra personal touch, put a drop of essential oil onto the envelope just before posting.

Presents
Scraps of pretty material and ribbon can make lovely pot-pourri bags for your friends (see 'Bedlinen' page 247). When wrapping presents, put a drop or two of essential oil onto the wrapping paper or the decorative bow.

Car
On a long journey it is essential to stay alert while driving and essential oils of lemon, rosemary and peppermint are efficient here. Special car vaporizers can be purchased (see Useful Addresses) or you can put the oils onto a kitchen tissue or ball of cotton wool, lodging it near an air stream (if you are driving and have a cold, substitute eucalyptus or black pepper for rosemary).

When you clean the inside of the car, use a damp cloth rinsed in water containing essential oils and spray freshening essential oils inside afterwards (diluted in water).

Smelly Shoes

Many people suffer from smelly feet; no matter how scrupulous they are with washing and frequent sock changing, their shoes end up with an unwanted odour. Spray them lightly every day when you take your shoes off (if you change into slippers when you get home, these can be sprayed just before you leave for work in the morning), making a mix of the oils given above for deodorizing hotel rooms.

Have a footbath every night and apply the same essential oils in a lotion or vegetable oil every morning after washing.

Pets

Pet lovers do not give much thought to the possibility of catching germs from their pets. Domestic animals can wander into many unsavoury situations and places, and are welcomed back into the kitchen, often without having their paws wiped unless they have been in the rain, and your floors are at risk. In some kitchens pets are even free to roam the worktops – not a good idea!

When your pet has its daily brushing, dampen the bristles in a basin of water containing three to four drops of tea tree oil; wipe paws with a cloth squeezed out in the same solution; add essential oils to the rinsing water after shampooing. Most animals love aromatherapy and we have many cases of arthritic dogs (and a budgerigar!), bronchial horses, and even cows with mastitis being helped by essential oils.

If your pet has fleas, add two drops red thyme and three drops tea tree to a cup of water and spray on to your pet (get a friend to keep a hand over the eyes and mouth); brush well and repeat as necessary. For a dog, the oils can be added to the shampoo and the rinsing water.

The same recipes as for a human being can be used on large animals, halving the quantities for small ones. For a cat, whose physiology is different from other domestic pets, the amount of essential oil used should be divided by five.[164]

Cooking with Essential Oils

Vegetables

When cooking cauliflower, after bringing my water to the boil and before adding the cauliflower, I add two to three drops of nutmeg essential oil – it completely kills the cooking smell, without noticeably flavouring the cauliflower (for this four to six drops would be needed). I do the same with cabbage, except that as I cook this by the conservation method, with very little water, one drop is sufficient. To give flavour, use two drops of bitter orange oil in carrots (using the conservation method again – delicious!), one drop of fennel in the sauce accompanying cauliflower – there are many other possible vegetable ideas!

Apple Pie
I add two drops of clove bud (or cinnamon) to about two tablespoons of water, gently cooking the apples in it, together with the sugar, and leave to cool while making the pastry. It is great to have the flavour without the actual cloves!

Cakes
You can vary the essential oils according to the cake – lemon, orange, spice loaf, etc. but the principle is the same. I put two to three drops of the essential oil (onto a teaspoon first, in case I get more than three drops) adding this to the eggs before beating them – after which I carry on as normal.

Soups
Essential oils can be used in soups instead of fresh herbs, if these are unavailable. Dried herbs do not retain their full flavour for long and the addition of essential oils as well gives enhanced flavour. Home-made soup is easy to make, tastes much better than dried or tinned soup and is very economical on the purse strings!

Len makes our soup, waiting until it is nearly finished before adding his oil of marjoram, basil, rosemary, black pepper etc. – or a blend of one or two. He always puts them first into a cup containing about a tablespoonful of water – one or two drops for three to four people, three to four drops for a party panful. He then adds a little of this to the soup and tastes it (very important), adding more if needed. Never hold the essential oil bottle over the pan – you may get more drops than you bargained for and ruin your soup!

Stir Fry and Curry
A drop of caraway oil in a stir fry adds a delicate extra flavour and Len puts two drops of ginger and one of black pepper in a mild curry to make it a little more exotic.

Salads (Fruit and Vegetable)

I often enhance a fruit salad by the use of petitgrain; mixing one drop in a tablespoonful of water first, I add a bit at a time to the juice I have made, tasting it before pouring it over the fruit. I use lemon oil if the salad juice is too sweet – and orange is another possibility. Orange flower water is delicious in a fruit salad (as is a teaspoonful in black coffee!)

A savoury dish I do like making is a vegetable salad. I have two small basins each containing three or four items (choose any four you like!), e.g. grated carrot, pine nuts, chopped black olives and currants; diced avocado, peach (or apple), mushrooms and pumpkin or sunflower seeds or perhaps diced red pepper, apple, cucumber and walnuts – there are many combinations. The lettuce, together with chopped parsley or dill and perhaps some bean sprouts or alfalfa goes into another bowl. I then make a salad dressing, separate it into three, adding one drop of a different essential oil to each, such as sweet fennel, caraway, sweet marjoram, basil, etc., before adding to the salads. I keep any dressing left over for next time, mixing all three together.

This year in France I was invited to a dinner cooked by an aromatherapy group from Germany. It was delicious – it included trout with essential oil of dill in the sauce; but the pièce de resistance was the lavender ice cream! What a delicate flavour! If you make your own ice cream it is definitely worth trying.

I could fill a whole book with cooking ideas, but I am sure that once you try the above, you will be able to use your imagination and use essential oils in stews, vegetable and meat lasagnes, etc. just as we do.

Points to Note when Cooking with Essential Oils

1. Remember, essential oils are concentrated.
2. Never add them directly to your cooking from the bottle – put onto a spoon or into a cup with water first.
3. Mix thoroughly into a liquid such as oil, water, sauce, eggs, etc.
4. Use **small quantities** – you can always add more, if required.

13 *Aromatherapy: Definition, Qualifications and Finding a Good Aromatherapist*

The definition of aromatherapy is assumed by most people to be 'a massage using essential oils'. It would be a little strong to say that nothing could be further from the truth, but this definition is only one-fifth of the story. Aromatherapy was being (and still is) practised in France without massage long before this concept was introduced. Also, massage is a therapy in its own right, enjoying success without employing essential oils and in massage, essential oils are an 'extra', not fundamental to the results.

Strictly speaking, aromatherapy means 'a therapy of aromas', and an expanded definition could be as follows; 'the (controlled) use of essential oils to maintain and promote the health and vitality of the spirit, the emotions and the physical body'.[165] This incorporates many practical methods of application, such as inhalation, baths, compresses, self-application *and* massage.

In Britain, since December 1992, doctors can refer their patients to a complementary therapist under the NHS, so long as the doctor remains in control of the patient. This is looked on as a very positive step forward. In Switzerland, Germany and France no-one who does not hold either a medical or health practitioner qualification (this last varies from country to country) is allowed to advertise or practise using the word 'therapy'. In Britain, we are under Common Law and can do whatever we like so long as we do not break the law, whereas most of Europe is under Napoleonic Law, where people can do nothing unless it is approved by the law. A new word is therefore being chosen in the rest of Europe to replace 'aromatherapy', and a whole new concept has arisen.

Len and I were present at a meeting in Zurich where the idea was first discussed by representatives of France, Germany and Switzerland. 'Osmology' was the first suggestion, rejected because it is already in use and, in any case, is more related to the study of smell. The second sugges-tion was 'aromatology'; this, beginning with 'aroma', would necessitate less explanation during the changeover period. An aromatology associa-tion has now been set up (the Institute of Aromatic Medicine) and the idea is a good one for three further reasons, as follows.

1. Aromatherapy Without Massage

From enquiries coming to our school it appears that by no means everyone wants either to learn, or to use essential oils with, massage – and the latter subject takes up a great deal of time (as indeed it should) in any aromatherapy course of note at the present time (where massage is part of the qualification obtained). At the moment, many nurses and qualified complementary therapists without aromatherapy qualifications are using essential oils without full knowledge of their potential benefits or possible hazards (see chapter 6), partly because they do not wish to attend a course where at least half of the study time is taken up with massage.

For such people a detailed course has been developed on essential oils (plus other factors related to the workings of the body in disease and health where required) and an Aromatology Certificate is awarded on completion. People qualified in, or currently studying, a recognized disci-pline (ranging from nursing or health counselling to acupuncture, osteopathy or medicine), can then utilize essential oils with full knowl-edge and complete confidence within their own discipline or therapy, in ways which do not necessarily include massage (other than perhaps hand, foot and shoulder) such as compresses, intensive application and internal use – which last requires a great deal of extra study on the essential oils. Those who wish to learn aromatherapy in conjunction with full body massage would continue to attend the present type of course – the essen-tial oil knowledge would be the same on each.

Aromatherapists wishing to increase their knowledge and qualify in aromatology or aromatic medicine would be exempt from those modules of the course in which they are already proficient.

2. Connotations of Aromatherapy

From being an almost unknown word a mere five or six years ago, aromatherapy is now on the tip of everyone's tongue. Chemists and gift shops sell aromatherapy bath oils, soaps and shampoos, and 'aroma' products are confused with therapeutic products. Second rate oils abound, making it difficult for the general public (and sometimes therapists) to know what they are buying; many oils are sold without suitable explanations being provided, either by leaflet or verbally by shop assistants. Newspaper and magazine articles grab the wrong end of the stick regarding 'toxicity' and frighten people away from the one thing they can utilize at home to improve their day-to-day health – and, in many cases, their happiness.

No-one, least of all myself, is suggesting that essential oils can be used carelessly or extravagantly, but as the majority of people use aspirins, bleach and vitamins (an excess of these can cause a health disaster!) in a sensible fashion, essential oils should not be treated any differently. More people die from over-use of alcohol and cigarettes than have been even off-colour from the use of essential oils.

It is sad that some officials and lay people in the church believe aromatherapy to be not of God, simply because essential oils are used by 'new age' disciplines like crystal healing and dowsing, which the church cannot understand – yet. Nevertheless, just because essential oils can be used with any discipline, *aromatherapy* should not be accredited with being 'part of' that particular discipline: aromatherapy is a separate discipline, complete in itself. The oils are natural products, from Nature's own plants so they are surely nearer to God than synthetic drugs, of which the church approves!

3. Qualifications

Many people attend a one or two day 'course' in aromatherapy (including some massage) to enable them to help themselves at home. The danger is that some begin to offer advice. As a result, those receiving such unqualified advice may not benefit as expected and may come away thinking aromatherapy is a load of rubbish, or even dangerous! There are many short courses which do not come up to the standards required by the professional organizations. I have talked to several people who have 'tried' aromatherapy and been disappointed. Their amazement at the difference in results is very apparent when persuaded to visit a fully trained therapist who may have spent anything from three months (full-time) to 12 or more months (part-time) learning about the essential oils, the workings of the body and full body massage. I am sometimes disheartened when I think of the people to whom I have not had the chance to speak. For this reason alone I feel it would be a good thing to have a new name for the therapy, even in Britain, which hopefully will not then be abused.

I am very pleased that some of these briefly 'trained' people are able to help their friends and relations with simple problems – some people have a natural healing gift with both touch and empathy. However, it is important that such people do not step beyond their sphere of knowledge and offer a general service to the public.

There is a possibility that you may find a well-trained therapist and still be unhappy. Qualified people in all walks of life are not necessarily 'good' at their job. They may excel in the theory, but be lacking in the practical application; lecturers, lawyers, teachers and practitioners of all disciplines may have no gift of communication (which is a severe handicap in a job which demands empathy). Fortunately, such people are few and far between and I can only hope that you find your aromatherapist from the vast majority of sincere, talented and genuine lovers of their art.

Some therapists possess certificates and others diplomas. Some people feel that a certificate is of a lesser standing than a diploma. This is erroneous: it is the course studied which determines the standing, not the name given to it. The City and Guilds teaching certificate (730) requires almost two years of part-time study; a friend of mine received a teaching *diploma* from a private college after only three months' part-time study; I studied for three years *full time* to become a teacher and received a certificate!

On a government-recognized teacher training course it was stated that the basic difference between certificates and diplomas was that certificates are awarded after part-time training and diplomas after full-time training. There was no officially recognized difference in standard, e.g. a certificate may indicate a higher standard of achievement than a diploma, or vice versa.

As in everything, it is the quality which counts, not the feeling about the name. The important thing is to find out whether or not the certificate (or diploma) held is one of course attendance only. An examination recognized by a leading body is essential; 'attendance' usually indicates short, incomplete training.

All aromatherapy associations and training establishments of note belong to the Aromatherapy Organisations Council (AOC), the regulating body for the therapy, formed in 1990 to unify the profession. One of its main functions is to set minimum standards for, and to represent, all associations and schools in aromatherapy and, at the time of writing, several thousand aromatherapists belong to it through their association or school.

The umbrella organization to which the AOC belongs is the British Complementary Medicine Association, the formation of which was a great step forward for all branches of complementary therapy. It was set up in response to the government's request (through the Parliamentary Group for Alternative and Complementary Medicine), for complementary therapies to 'get their house in order' and speak with a unified voice.

The Institute of Complementary Medicine (ICM) is also an umbrella organization for complementary therapies.

Finding a Good Aromatherapist

The definition of an aromatherapist in Britain is 'a therapist qualified in both the theory of essential oils and massage' and about 99 per cent of aromatherapists give treatments which include massage.

Training in Britain has always tied the two together and they do make a perfect pair, especially for disorders springing from an emotional source such as stress. Massage relaxes the body (when well done) and essential oils (which enter the body more quickly when it is relaxed) supply the therapeutic effects. If, however, you wish to have only a consultation with advice on how to help yourself at home (and no massage), make this clear when you arrange an appointment and a good aromatherapist will respect your wishes, and greet you courteously and caringly on arrival, possibly suggesting a 'prescription' after an assessment of your health.

The surest way of finding a good therapist is to have one recommended, from personal experience. Otherwise, a few questions when making the appointment could be a valuable aid. Ask if he or she is a member of an aromatherapy association. Your therapist should be aware of the AOC, and the association to which he or she belongs (or the school at which he/she completed training), should be a member of it.

Each member of an association is required to hold insurance for carrying out treatments on the general public and for using and mixing essential oils. Should you wish to visit a therapist who does not belong to an aromatherapy or aromatic medicine association, check that he or she is at least insured (perhaps through another therapy which is practised).

As the whole point of a professional aromatherapy or aromatology treatment is to have oils selected for you personally, it is important to ask whether a selection of individual oils, or ready mixed oils, will be used; for full therapeutic benefit individually selected oils should be used.

To summarize:

a) check that the certificate or diploma states that an examination has been taken – a certificate of attendance is not enough.
b) check that the therapist belongs to a professional association.
c) during the consultation, you should feel that the therapist is trying to find the cause of your problems, not treating the symptoms alone.
d) make sure that the therapist will be selecting individual oils for your treatment – not using a ready-made mix.

Holistic Health and Aromatherapy

Anybody can enjoy the benefits of an aromatherapy treatment from a qualified aromatherapist, but it is worth finding a really good one. The following is a guideline on what to expect from a good treatment. The therapist should:

a) greet you courteously and caringly, even on the phone.
b) explain what aromatherapy is, and the benefits it can give.
c) spend at least half an hour asking questions and noting down the answers. Most will use the reflexes of the feet to organize their questions and make it more interesting for you.
d) spend some minutes checking on the essential oils she/he has decided would be the most effective ones for your case, bearing in mind the symptoms manifested by the cause of your particular stress. This is very important. For a holistic treatment it is essential that the oils used are not ready mixed but selected especially for *you* (not entirely by memory or intuition but also by careful reference to the therapeutic manual, index or cross reference chart given to them on their training, to check the best possible combination for you).
e) give you a choice of the treatment method best suited to your problem, e.g. self-application, baths, inhalation, compresses (all to be carried out at home), or a professional massage.

If massage is chosen, it should be a wonderfully relaxing, smooth, rhythmical massage of part of, or your whole body (see chapter 10). It should be firm but not heavy, and a complete treatment will include not just the back and the legs but also the arms, scalp, face and chest and the abdomen.

f) advise you how you can continue the treatment at home, to be sure of the best and quickest results.

Aromatherapy Consultation

Ideally, every practitioner should have an accurate and detailed understanding not only of the anatomy of the human body but also of its physiological processes and functions. Without such knowledge any attempt at assessment of any sort is impossible.

A minimum of 30 minutes is usually allowed for an assessment, evaluation and analysis of a client. This initial meeting is very important as it allows the practitioner to determine, as far as is possible, the underlying cause of the symptoms; it gives the client time to relax and to build up a feeling of trust with the practitioner (who is there specifically to help). During this time, the practitioner will be deciding exactly what form the treatment should take; compresses, shoulder or back massage, home treatment only, a full aromatherapy body massage or Swiss reflex treatment (an effective aromatherapy treatment on the feet, devised by myself while in Switzerland – hence the name – and taught to all who take our Bodywork Certificate Course).

Some practitioners conduct only the consultation and assessment at the first appointment (carrying out any clinic treatment which may be indicated at a subsequent date), recommending home treatment there and then, if this is the best course of action.

Case-taking begins the moment the client enters the room. A lot can be learned from an initial handshake; whether it is hot or cold, wet or dry, firm or limp. The aromatherapist will be aware of many characteristics in the client; how the client walks, stands or sits; shoulder droop; fatness or thinness; skin colour; eyes; whether he or she is timid or aggressive; etc. In other words, the therapist is using his or her eyes to observe anything out of balance or different from the expected. The therapist will also listen to the breathing (is it quiet, noisy, laboured, etc.?) and the strength of voice (is it loud and firm, soft and hesitant?) Much can be learned, or verified, by a physical examination; stance, spine alignment, dry skin, overweight, water retention, etc. – all these are very important to the final picture.

This initial observation is followed by carefully phrased questions, often in conjunction with using the foot reflexes. This is not a reflexology treatment but simply a method of ensuring that every relevant fact concerning the client's health is thoroughly checked and noted down. An accomplished therapist is a good listener, and will be able to discover not only the fact that there is a digestive problem, but also that it is worse in the morning, the client feels sick after a meal, or has diarrhoea every now and then, etc. Through listening carefully to answers like 'It seems to happen a lot before my evening class' further questions can reveal why this is so. 'What subject is your evening class?', or 'Do you have to do something in front of the class?' etc.

In other words, a skilled therapist will listen, support, encourage and help clients to become aware of why or how they came to be ill, so that they can make their own decisions and recognize how they can help themselves. A proficient therapist will not do all the talking or 'take on' the client's problems; he or she will be empathetic (be able to appreciate and understand these problems), rather than sympathetic ('feeling sorry' for the client's situation).

Essential Oil Selection

The therapist will correlate all the information in such a way that specific essential oils may be selected. I believe that the therapist should refer to a manual while doing this. He or she will have to select from between 30 to 50 of the essential oils used in aromatherapy, and it is to the client's advantage that the oils to be used are selected for the specific effects required.

A few therapists work purely from intuition and, provided this is backed by adequate training, practical experimentation, appropriate experience and in-depth knowledge of essential oils, I have no quarrel with it. However, if I were a client I would be happier if such a therapist referred to an index (as mentioned earlier) to confirm any decision which may be made.

If the client has a particular skin condition and the treatment involves massage or home application, the carrier oil into which the essential oils are diluted will be chosen with this in mind. Much thought is put into the mix, which is individually tailored to a client's needs – be they mental, emotional, physical, bactericidal, etc. or, more usually, a combination.

Aromatherapy Body Massage

Full body massage completely relaxes the mind as well as the body and efficiently begins the removal of toxins – an important part of the treatment. Aromatherapy massage includes pressures down the spine, and some lymph drainage, and is carried out on the back, legs and arms, scalp, face (including the upper chest) and abdomen, giving a very thorough boost to both the blood and the lymphatic circulation (see chapter 10).

The deepest feeling of relaxation occurs during massage of the back, and as it is important for the success of the whole treatment that the body is as relaxed as possible, a full treatment should commence with this part of the body. Massage of the back of the legs usually follows, after which the client will be asked to turn over (which he or she usually does very reluctantly!) The treatment continues with massage of the front of the legs and the feet, working up the body to finish with final massage movements on the scalp. Obviously there will be slight variations (depending on the school attended by the therapist), but the principles of the massage should be the same (see chapter 10).

Some therapists then give an extra treatment on the face (if there are any unwelcome symptoms showing themselves, such as dry patches, sallow skin or acne). Apart from the benefit to the facial skin and adding a finishing touch enjoyed by most clients, it gives the client seven or eight minutes towards the time needed for the body rhythms to return to normal.

Conclusion

As the essential oils commence their journey around the body within the first ½ hour, it is safe to assume that whatever proportion is going to be absorbed through the skin has almost 'made it' by the time the final scalp massage has been accomplished. As it is better for the body not to exhale before the oils have taken hold, the client should not, after an aromatherapy massage, take a bath, sauna or shower until a few hours have elapsed.

If the therapist has used the right amount of oil for each part of the body, the skin (when the treatment is finished) should not feel oily or in need of a 'rinse' because of any oiliness.

It is possible (but by no means inevitable) that a client with a lot of toxins in the body may feel tired the next day, have a headache or diarrhoea. This is Nature's reaction to the release of some toxins into the body fluid. Should this occur (and it is rare), treatments in close succession, i.e. with a three or four day gap, will ensure that further toxins are removed quickly, so that the benefits accrue in a shorter period of time. If it is known that the client has a very toxic system, it may be advisable to massage only the legs, arms, shoulders and face, to slow down the exchange of toxins from the reticulo-endothelial system, where an overload of toxins is stored, back into the blood circulation (see chapter 9). It is the release of these into the general system which may make a few people feel slightly unwell after a full massage treatment.

Happily, most people immediately feel much better, continuing to improve over the next three or four days (especially with advised home treatment and further aromatherapy treatments), until the problem is no longer a major one. Should clients not be offered advice, I trust they will ask for it (they would not expect to leave an allopathic surgery without it!)

It is up to the client to carry out any advice given; cutting out certain types of food or drink and/or including something with extra nourishment (see chapter 9); putting oils into the bath or applying them onto parts of the body; attending a further appointment or being referred to a different therapy, should it be thought to be of benefit.

It may be necessary to visit the toilet after the treatment as the excretory system is stimulated; many therapists offer a cup of herbal tea or a glass of water to replace lost liquid, helping the body to maintain its stability for the journey home. If the client is driving, this rest period is important, as the relaxing effect of the treatment could make reflex actions, such as braking, slower (as with alcohol intake).

CASE EXAMPLE

Mr A, who had a nasty stye, was depressed and found himself snapping at his wife and children for no reason. He had recently changed to a more financially rewarding job – one which he said he enjoyed very much.

During the listening session, it appeared that his new employers found him such a good salesman that they asked him to lecture at sales meetings every now and then. He was coping quite well with this, but it was clearly not a task he relished. The medication from the doctor would not clear his stye (which usually recurred just before or just after sales meetings) and this upset him, as his job involved meeting people.

By piecing together the results of the consultation I could see that his problems were stress orientated. He was not keen to be massaged (he had never had a massage before), but I persuaded him to have one two days before his next sales talk the following week. Meanwhile I gave him my chamomile eye drops to help relieve the irritation caused by the stye.

When he returned, he admitted that he had come only because his eye had responded well to the drops, giving him the confidence to try a massage. Halfway through massaging his back (using two drops each of Roman chamomile and sweet marjoram and one drop of lavender) he relaxed and accepted this new experience. He telephoned three weeks later to make another appointment two days before his next lecture (in five weeks' time), telling me how relaxed he had felt during the lecture following his treatment. Also, his stye had not reappeared.

At his third treatment I learned that his wife had remarked on his happier frame of mind. He took home a mix of essential oils, to inhale and to put in the bath each night of the last few days before his lecture (instead of a treatment).

A year later he brought his daughter to see me regarding teenage acne and told me he was still benefiting from the oils, though he had had to buy a bigger bottle to share with his wife, because she loved the aroma!

Here we see someone who thought he was able to cope with the occasional lecture, but had bottled up the apprehension until it showed itself as a stye. Once there, apprehension became stress and this, together with his dislike of meeting people whilst suffering an inflamed eye, had made him depressed and consequently irritable with his family.

This case example is one of many which illustrate the importance of looking at the whole person, whatever the therapy discipline.

My aim in writing this book was to give readers a deeper insight into the effectiveness of essential oils and a broader knowledge of how to use them. Essential oils are filling more and more people with enthusiasm and 'addiction' such as I have experienced for the last 23 years (and still do!) and I trust we will all continue to learn, and to derive delight from their benefits.

14 *Therapeutic Uses of Essential Oils – Reference*

Therapeutic Effects of Essential Oils

The following list was compiled from several of the most reliable reference books available, plus the author's own experience. The oils in **bold** are the ones which occurred the most frequently in connection with the particular ailment.

ABDOMINAL CRAMP	Aniseed; **Basil**; Bergamot; Caraway; Clove bud; Fennel; Marjoram, sweet; **Melissa, true**; Nutmeg; Orange, bitter.
ABSCESSES/BOILS	Cajuput; **Chamomile, German**; Clove bud; Lavender; **Lemon**; **Niaouli**; Savory; Tea tree (infection); **Thyme, red** (infection); **Thyme, sweet**
ACNE	Benzoin; Cajuput; Chamomile, German; **Cedarwood**; Clove bud; **Geranium**; **Juniper berry**; Lavender; Neroli; Orange, bitter; Patchouli; **Petitgrain**; Rosemary; Thyme, sweet; Vetiver
AIR DISINFECTANT	Eucalyptus; Grapefruit; Lemon; **Pine**; Sage
ALLERGIES	Eucalyptus; Hyssop; Patchouli
ANTI-AGEING	Clary; **Frankincense**; **Geranium**; Lavender; Marjoram, sweet; **Neroli**; Orange, bitter; Patchouli; Parsley; **Rose Otto**; Rosewood; Vetiver; Ylang ylang
ANXIETY	**Basil**; Bergamot; Cedarwood; Chamomile, Roman; **Clary**; **Geranium**; **Lavender**; Lemon; **Marjoram, sweet**; Melissa, true; Myrrh; Neroli; Orange, sweet; Patchouli; Petitgrain; Rose Otto; Rosewood; Thyme, sweet; Valerian; Vetiver; Ylang ylang

APPETITE, LACK OF	Bergamot; Chamomile, Roman; **Coriander**; Fennel; Mandarin
ARTHRITIS	**Black Pepper**; **Cajuput**; Chamomile, German (inflammation); Chamomile, Moroccan; Chamomile, Roman; Clove bud; Coriander; Cypress; Frankincense; **Juniper**; Lavandin; Lavender; **Lemon**; Marjoram, sweet; Niaouli; **Sage**; Savory; **Thyme, sweet**
ASTHMA	**Aniseed**; Cajuput; Chamomile, Roman (nervous); Dill; **Eucalyptus**; Frankincense; **Hyssop**; Lavender; Lemon; Mandarin (difficult breathing); Niaouli; **Pine**; Rose Otto; Sage; Thyme, sweet
ATHLETE'S FOOT	Lavandin; Peppermint (refreshing); **Pine**; **Tagetes**; Tea tree
BAD BREATH	Basil; Bergamot; Caraway; Grapefruit; Lemon; Myrrh; Nutmeg; Orange, bitter; Thyme, sweet
BED WETTING	Cypress; Rosemary
BRONCHITIS	**Aniseed**; Black pepper; Cajuput; Cedarwood; Clove bud; **Cypress**; Eucalyptus; Frankincense; Ginger; **Hyssop**; Juniper; **Lavandin**; Lemon; Marjoram, Spanish; Marjoram, sweet; Myrrh; **Niaouli**; **Pine**; Rose Otto; Sage; Savory; Tea tree; Thyme, red; Thyme, sweet
BRUISES	Camphor; Chamomile, German; Fennel; **Hyssop**; **Marjoram, sweet**; Myrrh; Rosemary; Sage
BURNS	Benzoin; Chamomile, German; **Geranium**; **Lavender**; Sage
CANDIDA (THRUSH)	Bergamot; Cinnamon bark; Eucalyptus; Rosemary; Rose Otto; Rosewood; **Sage**; Tagetes; **Tea tree**; **Thyme, sweet**
CATARRH	Benzoin; Black Pepper; Cajuput; Cedarwood; Lemon; **Marjoram, Spanish**; Marjoram, sweet; **Niaouli**; Peppermint; Rosemary; Sage; Tagetes
CELLULITE	Cedarwood (lymph); Cypress; Geranium; Lemongrass (tone); Patchouli (congestion); Rosemary; Sage (congestion); Sandalwood (lymph)
CIRRHOSIS	Juniper; Rosemary
CONSTIPATION	Basil; Black Pepper; Chamomile; Coriander; Fennel; Ginger; Mandarin (gentle); Orange, bitter; **Rosemary**
COUGHS AND COLDS	Black Pepper; Cedarwood; Cypress; Eucalyptus; Geranium; Juniper; Lavender; Lemon; Marjoram, Spanish; Marjoram, sweet; Peppermint; Pine; Thyme, sweet (also see catarrh)

CRAMP

Basil; Cajuput; Chamomile, Roman (soothing); Cypress; Lavender; Mandarin (mild action); **Marjoram, sweet**; **Rosemary**; Valerian (sedative)

CUTS/WOUNDS

Benzoin; Bergamot; Camphor; Cedarwood; **Chamomile, German**; Clove bud (analgesic); Cypress; Frankincense; **Geranium** (bleeding); Hyssop; **Lavender**; Lemon; Myrrh; **Niaouli**; Orange, bitter; Rose Otto; **Rosemary**; Sage; Tea tree (infected)

CYSTITIS

Basil, sweet; Cajuput; Chamomile, German; Clove bud; Coriander; Eucalyptus; Hyssop; **Juniper**; Niaouli; Peppermint; **Sandalwood**; Thyme, red; Thyme, sweet

DEBILITY

Basil; Camphor; Cinnamon bark; Clove bud; **Coriander**; Geranium; Hyssop; **Lavandin**; **Marjoram, sweet**; Peppermint; Pine; Rosewood; Savory; Tea tree; Thyme, red; **Thyme, sweet**; Valerian

DEPRESSION

Basil; Chamomile, Moroccan; Cinnamon bark; Cypress; Frankincense; Geranium; **Hyssop**; Juniper; Lavender; Marjoram, sweet; **Neroli**; Niaouli; **Petitgrain**; **Pine**; Rosemary; Rose Otto; Rosewood; **Sandalwood**; Tea tree; **Thyme, red**; **Thyme, sweet**; Vetiver; Ylang ylang

DERMATITIS

Benzoin; Bergamot; Cajuput; **Chamomile, German**; **Chamomile, Moroccan** (dry); Eucalyptus (bacterial); **Geranium**; Hyssop; **Juniperberry**; Lavender; Patchouli; Rose Otto; Sage; Thyme, sweet

DIABETES

Clary; Eucalyptus; Geranium; Juniper; **Lemon**; Pine; Thyme, red; **Thyme, sweet**; **Vetiver**; Ylang ylang

DIARRHOEA

Chamomile, Roman; Cinnamon bark; Clove bud; Geranium; **Ginger**; Juniper; Lemon; Marjoram, sweet; Myrrh; Niaouli; Nutmeg; **Peppermint**; Sandalwood; Savory

EARACHE

Basil; Cajuput (inflammation); Chamomile, Roman; Lavender; Rosemary

ECZEMA

Basil (dry); Benzoin; Cajuput; **Chamomile, German** (irritation); **Chamomile, Moroccan**; Clove bud; Eucalyptus; Frankincense (weeping); **Geranium**; Hyssop (weeping); **Juniper**; **Lavender**; Myrrh (weeping); Niaouli (weeping); Patchouli (weeping); Rose Otto; Sandalwood (dry); Thyme, sweet (dry)

EPILEPSY	Basil; Cajuput; Clary; Lavender; Marjoram, sweet; Parsley leaf; Rosemary; Thyme, sweet
FLATULENCE	**Aniseed**; **Basil**; Bergamot; **Caraway**; **Coriander**; **Fennel**; Ginger; Lavender; Mandarin; Marjoram, sweet; Niaouli; Orange, bitter; **Peppermint**; **Thyme, sweet**
FLU	Clove bud; Coriander; **Eucalyptus**; Lavandin; Myrrh; **Niaouli**; Peppermint; **Pine**; Rosemary; **Sage**; Tea tree; **Thyme, sweet**
FLUID RETENTION	**Cedarwood**; Cypress; **Geranium** (congestion); **Juniperberry**; Lavender; Rosemary (congestion)
FRIGIDITY	Aniseed; Black Pepper; Chamomile, Moroccan; Ginger; Pine; Rose Otto; Savory; Ylang ylang
FUNGAL INFECTIONS (SKIN)	Cypress; Geranium; Lavandin; Niaouli; Patchouli; Peppermint; Pine; Rosemary; Sage; Sandalwood; Savory; Tagetes; Tea tree; Thyme, sweet
GASTRIC ULCERS	Basil; **Chamomile, German**; **Geranium**; Lemon; Marjoram, sweet; Niaouli; Peppermint
GASTROENTERITIS	**Basil** (spasm); Bergamot; **Cajuput**; Caraway (spasm); **Chamomile, German**; Chamomile, Moroccan; Clove bud; Coriander; Cypress; Fennel; **Juniperberry**; Lavandin; Lemongrass; Mandarin; Marjoram, sweet; **Niaouli**; Nutmeg; Patchouli; **Peppermint**; Sage; Tea tree (virus); **Thyme, red** (virus); **Thyme, sweet**
GINGIVITIS	Clary; Juniper; Lemon; Sage
GLANDULAR INFLAMMATION	**Geranium** (anti-inflammatory); Pine; Rosemary; **Sage**; Thyme, sweet
GOUT	Basil; Chamomile, Roman; Fennel; **Juniper**; Lemon; Pine; Rosemary
GUM INFECTIONS (PYORRHOEA)	Cinnamon bark; Clove bud; **Cypress**; **Geranium**; **Juniperberry**; **Rosemary**; Tea tree
HAEMORRHOIDS	Bergamot; Cajuput; **Clary**; **Cypress**; Frankincense (healing); Geranium; Myrrh (inflammation); **Neroli**; **Niaouli**; Patchouli; Sandalwood (soothing); Tea tree; Valerian
HEADACHE	Chamomile, Roman; Eucalyptus (congestive); **Lavender**; Lemon; **Marjoram, sweet**; Melissa, true; Peppermint (digestive); Rosemary
HEARTBURN	Chamomile, Moroccan; Chamomile, Roman; Peppermint; Sandalwood

HEPATITIS	Basil; Clove bud; Eucalyptus; Juniper; Lemongrass; Myrrh; Niaouli; Petitgrain; Rosemary
HERPES	Bergamot; Eucalyptus; Geranium; Lavender; Lemon; Niaouli (genital); Sage
HICCUPS	Mandarin
HIGH BLOOD PRESSURE	Basil, sweet; Juniper (diuretic); **Lavender**; **Lemon**; **Marjoram, sweet**; **Ylang ylang** (Never stop allopathic treatment without advice)
HORMONAL OILS	See Table 9 (page 276)
HYSTERIA	Lemongrass; **Melissa, true**
IMMUNOSTIMULANT OILS	See Table 9 (page 276)
IMPOTENCE	Aniseed; Black Pepper; Cinnamon bark; **Ginger**; Peppermint; Pine (stimulates sperm production); Rose Otto; Savory; Thyme, sweet; **Ylang ylang**
INDIGESTION	**Aniseed**; Basil (nervous); Bergamot; Black Pepper; Caraway; **Coriander**; Dill; **Fennel**; **Ginger**; **Lemon**; Lemongrass; Mandarin; Melissa, true; Orange, bitter; Orange, sweet (children); **Peppermint**; Rosemary
INFLAMMATION	Chamomile, German; Clary; Frankincense; Geranium; Lavender; Myrrh; Peppermint (no more than 1%); Rose Otto; Sandalwood
INSECT BITES	Basil; Cajuput; Lavender; Melissa, true; Niaouli; Sage; Tea tree; Thyme, sweet
INSECT REPELLENT	Basil; Cedarwood; Clove bud; **Eucalyptus**; **Geranium**; Lemon; Peppermint
INSOMNIA	Bergamot; Chamomile, Roman; Cypress; Geranium; **Lavender**; Lemon; Mandarin; **Marjoram, sweet**; **Melissa, true**; Neroli; Orange, bitter; Orange, sweet; Rose Otto; Sandalwood; Valerian; Ylang ylang
IRRITATION (SKIN)	**Chamomile, German**; Cedarwood; Lavender; Neroli; Peppermint (no more than 1%); **Sandalwood**
KIDNEY, GENERAL	Cedarwood; Eucalyptus; Fennel; Geranium; Juniper; Lavender; Lemon; Niaouli; Pine; Sage; Sandalwood; Thyme, red; Thyme, sweet
KIDNEY INFECTIONS	Clove bud; Coriander; Myrrh; **Sandalwood**; Sage; Savory; **Thyme, red**; **Thyme, sweet**
KIDNEY STONES	Fennel; Geranium; Hyssop; Juniper; Lemon

LABOUR PAIN	Clary; Fennel; Nutmeg
LARYNGITIS	Black Pepper; Cajuput; Cypress; Eucalyptus; **Lemon**; Myrrh; Niaouli; Peppermint; **Sage**; Sandalwood (soothing)
LIVER, SLUGGISH	Basil*; Black Pepper; Cajuput; **Chamomile, Moroccan**; Juniper; **Lemon**; Lemongrass; Melissa, true; Peppermint*; **Rosemary***; **Thyme, sweet**; Vetiver (*also sluggish bile)
LOW BLOOD PRESSURE	Clove bud; Neroli; **Rosemary**; Savory; **Thyme, sweet**
LUMBAGO	Aniseed; Eucalyptus; Fennel; Geranium; Sandalwood
MENOPAUSE	Aniseed; Chamomile, Roman; **Clary**; Cypress; **Fennel**; Geranium; Lemon; Mandarin; Melissa, true; Peppermint (hot flush); Pine; **Rose Otto**; **Sage**; Sandalwood
MENTAL FATIGUE	**Basil**; Cajuput; **Clove bud**; Coriander; Juniperberry; Neroli; **Peppermint**; **Rosemary**; Rosewood
MIGRAINE	Aniseed (nausea); Basil; Chamomile, German; Eucalyptus; Marjoram, sweet (menstrual); Melissa, true; Peppermint; Rosemary
MILK, LACK OF (BREASTFEEDING)	Aniseed; Dill; Fennel
MOUTH ULCERS	Basil; Clove bud; Geranium; Juniper; Lemon; Myrrh; Niaouli; Rose Otto; Sage; Tea tree
MUSCULAR PAIN	**Black Pepper** (analgesic); Camphor; Chamomile, German; Chamomile, Moroccan; Chamomile, Roman; Frankincense; **Juniper**; **Nutmeg** (analgesic); **Rosemary**; **Thyme, sweet**; Vetiver
NAUSEA	Black Pepper; Caraway; Fennel; Ginger; Mandarin (pregnancy); Melissa, true; Peppermint (travel); Sandalwood (soothing)
NERVOUS EXHAUSTION	**Basil** (balancing); Clary; Clove bud; Coriander; Geranium; **Savory** (tonic); Tea tree; Thyme, sweet
NEURALGIA	Camphor; **Chamomile, Roman**; **Clove bud**; **Eucalyptus**; Ginger; **Juniperberry**; Lavandin; Marjoram, sweet; **Peppermint**; Pine; Rosemary; Sandalwood
NEURITIS	Chamomile, German; Chamomile, Roman; Clary; Cypress; Clove; Juniper; Niaouli; Thyme, sweet
OEDEMA	Cedarwood; Cypress; Geranium; **Juniper**
OSTEOPOROSIS	Eucalyptus; Lavender; Lemon; Lemongrass; Rosemary; Sage

OVARIES	Clary (stimulant); Cypress; Rosemary (regulator); Sage; Ylang ylang (stimulant)
PALPITATIONS	**Aniseed**; Fennel; Lavender; Mandarin; Melissa, true; **Neroli**; Petitgrain; **Rosemary**; Valerian; Ylang ylang
PERIODS, LACK OF	Aniseed; **Chamomile, German**; Cinnamon bark; **Clary**; **Fennel**; Peppermint (tonic); Rosemary; **Sage**; Tagetes; **Thyme, sweet**; Vetiver
PERIODS, PAINFUL	Aniseed; **Basil** (congestion); Chamomile, German (congestion); Clary; Cypress (congestion); Fennel; Geranium (congestion); Juniper; Marjoram, sweet; Peppermint; Pine; Sage (congestion)
PERIODS, SCANTY	**Chamomile, Roman**; Clary (hormonal); **Fennel**; Juniper; Lavender; **Melissa, true** (hormonal); Rosemary; **Rose Otto** (hormonal); Thyme, sweet
PERSPIRATION	Basil; Cypress; Geranium; Lavender; Neroli; Sage
PREMENSTRUAL SYNDROME	Chamomile, Roman; **Clary**; Geranium; Lavender; Melissa, true; Rose Otto; Neroli; Sage (congestion); Sandalwood
PROSTATE, ENLARGED	Basil; Caraway; Cypress
PSORIASIS	Benzoin; Bergamot; Cajuput; Lavender; Niaouli
RESPIRATORY INFECTION	Frankincense; Lemon; Niaouli; Petitgrain; Pine; Rosewood; Tagetes; Thyme, red
RHEUMATISM	**Basil**; Black Pepper; **Cajuput**; Camphor; Clove bud; **Eucalyptus**; Frankincense; Geranium (inflammation); **Ginger** (warming); Hyssop; **Juniper**; Lavandin; **Lavender**; Lemon (anti-inflammatory); Lemongrass; **Marjoram, sweet**; Myrrh; Niaouli; **Nutmeg** (analgesic); Petitgrain (nervous); Pine; **Rosemary** (stiffness); **Sage**; Savory; Thyme, sweet (tonic)
SCARS	Cedarwood; Frankincense; Hyssop; Lavender; Myrrh; Patchouli
SCIATICA	Camphor; **Chamomile, Roman**; Clove bud; **Eucalyptus**; Ginger; **Juniperberry**; Lavandin; Marjoram, sweet; **Peppermint**; Pine; Rosemary; Sandalwood
SHINGLES	**Clove bud**; Eucalyptus; Frankincense; **Geranium**; Niaouli; Peppermint; **Sage**; **Thyme, sweet**
SHOCK	Chamomile, Roman; Mandarin; Melissa, true; Neroli; Peppermint; Ylang ylang

SINUSITIS	Basil; Cajuput; **Clove bud**; **Eucalyptus**; Hyssop; Marjoram, Spanish; **Marjoram, sweet**; Niaouli; **Peppermint**; **Pine**; Rosemary; Sage; Tea tree; **Thyme, sweet**
SKIN, CRACKED/ CHAPPED	**Benzoin**; Chamomile, German; **Patchouli**; Rose Otto; Sandalwood
SKIN, DRY	**Chamomile, German**; Chamomile, Roman; Geranium; **Lavender**; **Neroli**; Petitgrain; Rose Otto; Sandalwood
SKIN, MATURE	Benzoin; **Clary**; **Fennel**; **Frankincense**; Lavender; Myrrh
SKIN, OILY (OPEN PORES)	Bergamot; Camphor; **Cedarwood**; **Cypress**; Geranium; **Juniper**; Lavender; Lemon; Ylang ylang
SKIN, SENSITIVE	Chamomile, German; Neroli; Rose Otto
SORE THROAT	**Cedarwood**; Clove bud; **Eucalyptus**; Geranium (inflammation); Lavender (inflammation); Lemon; Peppermint; Niaouli; **Sandalwood** (soothing); **Thyme, sweet**
SPRAINS	Hyssop; Lavender; Marjoram, sweet; Nutmeg (analgesic); Rosemary; Rose Otto
STIMULANT	Cypress; Marjoram, sweet; Niaouli
STRESS RELATED	Aniseed; Chamomile, Roman; Fennel; Marjoram, sweet; Petitgrain; Thyme, red; Thyme, sweet
STRETCH MARKS	Frankincense; Geranium; Lavender; Myrrh; Orange, bitter
SUNBURN	Geranium; Lavender; Peppermint (no more than 1%); Sandalwood
SWEATY SMELLS	Cypress; **Ginger**; **Nutmeg**; Pine; Sage; **Savory**; Thyme, red; Thyme, sweet
TENDONITIS	Chamomile, German; Chamomile, Roman; Frankincense; Juniperberry; Pine; Rosemary
THREAD VEINS	**Chamomile, German**; Chamomile, Roman; **Cypress**; Frankincense; Lavender; **Lemon**; **Neroli**; Orange, sweet; Patchouli; Peppermint; **Rose Otto**
THYROID, OVERACTIVE	Clove bud; Marjoram, sweet; Myrrh
TONIC (CIRCULATION)	Cedarwood (lymph); Cypress; Orange, bitter; Rosemary (blood); Sage; Sandalwood; Thyme, sweet
TONIC (MUSCLES)	Black Pepper; Cinnamon
TONSILLITIS	Clove bud; Eucalyptus; Geranium; **Lemon**; **Niaouli**; Rosemary; **Sage**; **Thyme, sweet**

TOOTHACHE	Black Pepper; Cajuput; Chamomile, Roman (teething); **Clove bud**; Ginger; Nutmeg; Pine; Sage
TRAVEL SICKNESS	Caraway; Ginger; Peppermint
ULCERS	Benzoin; Chamomile, German; Geranium; Lavender; Lemon; Myrrh
VAGINITIS	Chamomile, German; Clary; Lavender; Niaouli (infection); Tea tree (infection); Thyme, red (infection); Thyme, sweet
VARICOSE ULCERS	Benzoin; Chamomile, German; Geranium; Lavender; **Lemon; Myrrh; Niaouli**
VARICOSE VEINS	**Basil**; Cajuput; **Clary; Cypress**; Juniper (stimulation); Lemon; **Neroli; Niaouli**; Patchouli (decongestant); Peppermint (cooling); Rosemary (astringent); Sandalwood (soothing); Tea tree; Valerian
VERRUCAE	Lemon; Thyme, sweet
VERTIGO	**Caraway**; Fennel; Lavender; Lemon; Marjoram, sweet; **Melissa, true**; Orange, bitter
WRINKLES	Fennel; Frankincense; Neroli; Rose Otto

TABLE 9: Therapeutic Effects of Oils

	Analgesic	Anaphrodisiac	Anti-allergic	Anti-catarrhal	Anticoagulant	Antifungal	Anti-infectious	Anti-inflammatory	Antispasmodic	Antiviral	Astringent	Bactericidal	Balancing	Carminative	Cicatrizant
Aniseed* *(Pimpinella anisum)*	X	X							X			X		X	
Basil (sweet) *(Ocimum basilicum)*				X					X	X		X			X
Benzoin *(Styrax benzoin)*				X											X
Bergamot *(Citrus bergamia)*							X		X			X			X
Black Pepper *(Piper nigrum)*	X			X											
Cajuput *(Melaleuca leucadendron)*	X						X	X	X	X		X			
Camphor Wood *(Cinnamomum camphora)*	X			X											
Camphor Leaf *(Cinnamomum camphora)*						X	X			X		X			
Caraway *(Carum carvi)*				X					X					X	
Cedarwood *(Cedrus atlantica)*															
Chamomile, German *(Chamomilla recutita)*	X		X					X	X						X
Chamomile, Moroccan *(Ormenis mixta)*							X					X			
Chamomile, Roman *(Chamaemelum nobile)*								X	X						X
Cinnamon Bark* *(Cinnamomum zeylanicum)*	X						X	X		X		X			
Cinnamon Leaf* *(Cinnamomum zeylanicum)*							X	X		X		X			
Clary *(Salvia sclarea)*							X		X			X			
Clove Bud* *(Syzygium aromaticum)*	X						X	X		X		X			
Coriander *(Coriandrum sativum)*	X						X	X	X	X		X		X	
Cypress *(Cupressus semperivirens)*							X		X		X	X	X		
Dill *(Anethum graveolens)*															
Eucalyptus *(Eucalyptus globulus)*				X			X	X		X		X			
Fennel *(Foeniculum vulgare)*	X								X			X		X	
Frankincense *(Boswellia carteri)*	X			X					X				X		X
Geranium *(Pelargonium graveolens)*	X		X	X	X	X	X					X	X		X
Ginger *(Zingiber officinale)*	X			X										X	
Grapefruit *(Citrus paradisi)*															
Hyssop* *(Hyssopus officinalis)*			X	X	X		X	X		X		X			X
Juniper *(Juniperus communis)*											X		X		
Juniperberry *(Juniperus communis)*	X			X			X	X	X			X	X		
Lavandin *(Lavandula x intermedia)*				X		X				X		X			

* should not be available to the general public

Decongestant, gen.	Deodorant	Diuretic	Emmenagogic	Expectorant	Galactogogic	Hepatic	Hormonal	Hypertensive	Hypotensive	Immunostimulant	Lipolytic	Mucolytic	Parasiticide	Relaxant	Sedative	Stimulant, circ.	Stimulant, dig.	Tonic, digestion	Tonic, general	Tonic, nerve	Tonic, respiratory	Tonic, sexual
		X	X		X		X									X	X	X			X	
X		X				X								X		X	X	X	X			
			X																			
													X	X	X		X		X	X		
X				X												X	X					X
						X						X										
											X	X							X	X		
																			X			
											X	X				X						
													X		X	X						
X		X					X									X	X					
													X						X	X		
													X									
			X										X						X	X	X	X
								X	X			X	X						X	X		
				X									X							X		
						X	X			X			X		X	X			X	X		
													X			X			X	X		
	X												X						X	X		
												X				X	X					
				X								X										
		X	X	X		X										X	X	X			X	
				X						X				X					X	X		
				X											X	X		X	X			
X	X		X													X	X	X				X
		X														X	X					
			X	X									X						X			
		X	X												X	X					X	
																X						

	Analgesic	Anaphrodisiac	Anti-allergic	Anti-catarrhal	Anticoagulant	Antifungal	Anti-infectious	Anti-inflammatory	Antispasmodic	Antiviral	Astringent	Bactericidal	Balancing	Carminative	Cicatrizant
Lavender *(Lavandula angustifolia)*	X		X	X			X	X	X			X			X
Lemon *(Citrus limon)*							X	X		X	X	X	X	X	X
Lemongrass* *(Cymbopogon citratus)*							X								
Mandarin *(Citrus reticulata)*									X						
Marjoram, Spanish *(Thymus mastichina)*				X			X					X			
Marjoram, sweet *(Origanum majorana)*	X	X			X		X		X			X		X	
Melissa, true *(Melissa officinalis)*								X	X						
Myrrh *(Commiphora myrrha)*		X				X	X								X
Neroli *(Citrus aurantium v. amara* flos*)*							X					X	X		
Niaouli *(Melaleuca viridiflora)*	X			X			X	X		X		X	X		X
Nutmeg* *(Myristica fragrans)*	X													X	
Orange, bitter *(Citrus aurantium* v. *amara* per*)*				X					X						
Orange, sweet *(Citrus aurantium v. sinensis)*												X	X		
Patchouli *(Pogostemon patchouli)*						X	X	X							
Peppermint *(Mentha x piperita)*	X						X	X		X		X		X	
Petitgrain *(Citrus aurantium v. amara* fol*)*							X	X	X			X	X		
Pine *(Pinus sylvestris)*							X	X							
Rose otto *(Rosa centifolia)*							X				X				X
Rosemary *(Rosmarinus officinalis)*	X			X			X		X			X		X	X
Rosewood *(Aniba rosaeodora)*							X			X	X	X			X
Sage *(Salvia officinalis)*				X			X				X	X	X		X
Sandalwood *(Santalulm album)*												X			
Savory* *(Satureia montana)*	X						X				X	X			
Tagetes *(Tagetes glandulifera)*				X		X	X								
Tea Tree *(Malaleuca alternifolia)*	X						X	X	X	X		X			
Thyme* *(Thymus vulgaris* – phenols*)*							X					X			
Thyme, sweet *(Thymus vulgaris* – alcohols*)*						X	X			X		X			
Valerian *(Valeriana officinalis)*									X						
Vetiver *(Vetiveria zizanioides)*						X	X								
Ylang ylang *(Cananga odorata)*									X				X		

* should not be available to the general public

Decongestant, circ.	Decongestant, gen.	Deodorant	Diuretic	Emmenagogic	Expectorant	Galactogogic	Hepatic	Hormonal	Hypertensive	Hypotensive	Immunostimulant	Lipolytic	Mucolytic	Parasiticide	Relaxant	Sedative	Stimulant, circ.	Stimulant, dig.	Tonic, digestion	Tonic, general	Tonic, nerve	Tonic, respiratory	Tonic, sexual
										X					X	X				X			
			X				X								X		X	X	X				
																X		X	X				
															X								
					X																		
								X		X					X	X					X		
										X					X	X			X				
					X			X						X									
										X					X						X		
	X				X		X	X		X	X			X						X			
		X		X											X	X				X	X		
																X	X		X	X			
															X			X					
										X										X			
							X	X	X				X					X	X	X	X		
							X								X			X	X		X		
	X							X	X											X	X		
								X												X	X		X
			X		X		X	X					X							X			
														X						X			X
	X			X	X			X	X			X	X							X			
			X						X						X					X			X
									X		X			X				X		X			X
				X									X										
										X				X									
															X					X			
															X					X			
			X		X										X	X							
							X												X				
										X					X								X

TABLE 10: Therapeutic Reference Chart on the Uses of Essential Oils

DIGESTIVE

Essential Oil	Stimulating	Nausea	Liver, sluggish	Lack of Appetite	Indigestion	Gastric Ulcers	Gastro-enteritis	Flatulence	Diarrhoea	Diabetes	Constipation	Abdominal Cramp
Aniseed* (Pimpinella anisum)					X			X				X
Basil (sweet) (Ocimum basilicum)	X		X		X	X	X	X			X	X
Benzoin (Styrax benzoin)												
Bergamot (Citrus bergamia)							X	X				X
Black Pepper (Piper nigrum)	X	X	X				X					
Cajuput (Melaleuca leucadendron)	X	X	X				X					
Camphor Wood (Cinnamomum camphora)	X						X				X	
Caraway (Carum carvi)												
Cedarwood (Cedrus atlantica)										X		
Chamomile, German (Chamomilla recutita)							X				X	
Chamomile, Moroccan (Ormenis mixta)							X				X	
Chamomile, Roman (Chamaemelum nobile)												
Cinnamon Bark* (Cinnamomum zerum)									X			
Clary (Salvia sclarea)												
Clove Bud* (Syzygium aromaticum)					X	X	X	X	X		X	X
Coriander (Coriandrum sativum)					X		X		X		X	
Cypress (Cupressus sempervirens)							X					
Dill (Anethum graveolens)					X							
Eucalyptus (Eucalyptus globulus)												
Fennel (Foeniculum vulgare)		X	X	X	X		X	X	X		X	X
Frankincense (Boswellia carteri)												
Geranium (Pelargonium graveolens)					X			X	X	X		
Ginger (Zingiber officinale)	X	X										
Grapefruit (Citrus paradisi)												
Hyssop* (Hyssopus officinalis)												
Juniper (Juniperus communis)	X	X		X	X			X		X		
Juniperberry (Juniperus communis)	X	X		X	X			X		X		

CIRCULATION, MUSCLES, JOINTS

Essential Oil	Varicose Veins	Tonic (circ.)	Sprains	Rheumatism	Palpitations	Muscular Pain	Lumbago	LBP	HBP	Haemorrhoids	Gout	Fluid Retention	Cramp	Cellulite	Arthritis
Aniseed* (Pimpinella anisum)					X		X								
Basil (sweet) (Ocimum basilicum)	X			X					X		X		X		
Benzoin (Styrax benzoin)				X											X
Bergamot (Citrus bergamia)										X					
Black Pepper (Piper nigrum)	X			X		X					X				X
Cajuput (Melaleuca leucadendron)	X			X									X		X
Camphor Wood (Cinnamomum camphora)				X											
Caraway (Carum carvi)															
Cedarwood (Cedrus atlantica)		X									X		X		X
Chamomile, German (Chamomilla recutita)	X					X									X
Chamomile, Moroccan (Ormenis mixta)						X									X
Chamomile, Roman (Chamaemelum nobile)						X									X
Cinnamon Bark* (Cinnamomum zerum)								X							
Clary (Salvia sclarea)	X							X		X	X				X
Clove Bud* (Syzygium aromaticum)															X
Coriander (Coriandrum sativum)		X		X											X
Cypress (Cupressus sempervirens)	X	X								X		X	X	X	X
Dill (Anethum graveolens)												X			
Eucalyptus (Eucalyptus globulus)				X			X								
Fennel (Foeniculum vulgare)	X				X		X			X					
Frankincense (Boswellia carteri)				X		X	X			X					X
Geranium (Pelargonium graveolens)	X			X								X		X	X
Ginger (Zingiber officinale)				X		X									
Grapefruit (Citrus paradisi)												X		X	
Hyssop* (Hyssopus officinalis)				X											
Juniper (Juniperus communis)	X			X		X					X		X		X
Juniperberry (Juniperus communis)				X		X						X			

Oil																			
Lavandin (*Lavandula x intermedia*)	X									X		X	X							
Lavender (*Lavandula angustifolia*)	X	X	X							X	X		X							
Lemon (*Citrus limon*)	X		X		X	X				X	X									
Lemongrass* (*Cymbopogon citratus*)		X																		
Mandarin (*Citrus reticulata*)			X									X	X			X				
Marjoram, Spanish (*Thymus mastichina*)																				
Marjoram, sweet (*Origanum majorana*)	X	X			X						X	X	X	X						
Melissa, True (*Melissa officinalis*)										X						X	X			
Myrrh (*Commiphora myrrha*)												X				X				
Neroli (*Citrus aurantium v. amara flos*)				X	X					X										
Niaouli (*Melaleuca viridiflora*)	X			X	X					X		X	X			X	X			
Nutmeg* (*Myristica fragrans*)	X									X	X	X	X			X	X			
Orange, bitter (*Citrus aurantium v. amara per*)															X					
Orange, sweet (*Citrus aurantium v. sinensis*)															X					
Patchouli (*Pogostemon patchouli*)		X			X											X	X			
Peppermint (*Mentha x piperita*)										X	X					X	X			
Petitgrain (*Citrus aurantium v. amara fol*)																X	X			
Pine (*Pinus sylvestris*)			X						X											
Rose Otto (*Rosa centifolia*)																				
Rosemary (*Rosmarinus officinalis*)	X	X	X		X					X	X	X	X			X	X			
Rosewood (*Aniba rosaeodora*)																				
Sage (*Salvia officinalis*)	X	X								X						X				
Sandalwood (*Santalum album*)	X			X	X					X		X						X	X	
Savory* (*Satureia montana*)	X				X													X	X	
Tagetes (*Tagetes glandulifera*)																				
Tea Tree (*Melaleuca alternifolia*)																X	X			
Thyme* (*Thymus vulgaris* – phenols)															X	X	X			
Thyme, sweet (*Thymus vulgaris* – alcohols)	X		X		X					X		X	X			X	X			
Valerian (*Valeriana officinalis*)										X										
Vetiver (*Vetiveria zizanioides*)																		X	X	
Ylang ylang (*Cananga odorata*)		X								X		X	X			X	X			

* = should not be available to the general public

The following table is organised with two main categories down the left side — **NERVOUS** and **GENITO-URINARY** — each symptom forming a row, and essential oils forming the columns.

Category	Symptom	Aniseed* (Pimpinella anisum)	Basil (sweet) (Ocimum basilicum)	Benzoin (Styrax benzoin)	Bergamot (Citrus bergamia)	Black Pepper (Piper nigrum)	Cajuput (Melaleuca leucadendron)	Camphor Wood (Cinnamomum camphora)	Caraway (Carum carvi)	Cedarwood (Cedrus atlantica)	Chamomile, German (Chamomilla recutita)	Chamomile, Moroccan (Ormenis mixta)	Chamomile, Roman (Chamaemelum nobile)	Cinnamon Bark* (Cinnamomum verum)	Clary (Salvia sclarea)	Clove Bud* (Syzygium aromaticum)	Coriander (Coriandrum sativum)	Cypress (Cupressus sempervirens)	Dill (Anethum graveolens)	Eucalyptus (Eucalyptus globulus)	Fennel (Foeniculum vulgare)	Frankincense (Boswellia carteri)	Geranium (Pelargonium graveolens)	Ginger (Zingiber officinale)	Grapefruit (Citrus paradisi)	Hyssop* (Hyssopus officinalis)	Juniper (Juniperus communis)	Juniperberry (Juniperus communis)
NERVOUS	Vertigo							X																	X			
	Stress Related	X																					X					
	Shock																						X					
	Sciatica							X								X							X	X				X
	Neuralgia							X								X							X	X				X
	Nervous Exhaustion	X													X	X	X					X				X		
	Migraine	X	X										X									X						
	Mental Fatigue		X							X						X	X											X
	Insomnia				X								X						X			X						
	Impotence	X					X								X								X					
	Headache												X									X						
	Frigidity	X					X					X											X					
	Epilepsy		X				X							X														
	Depression		X								X			X							X							X
	Debility		X							X				X		X	X			X								X
	Anxiety		X		X							X	X		X					X	X							X
	Agitation				X							X	X							X	X							X
GENITO-URINARY	Vaginitis										X				X													
	PMS										X				X						X							
	Periods, Scanty										X				X			X			X						X	
	Periods, Painful	X	X								X				X			X			X						X	
	Periods, Lack of	X	X							X			X		X		X											
	Menopause	X	X										X		X						X							
	Labour Pain														X	X					X							
	Cystitis		X				X				X					X	X											X
	Candida (Thrush)			X										X						X								

*Oils marked with an asterisk (*) should be used with caution.

Essential Oil																				
Lavandin (Lavandula x intermedia)																		X	X	
Lavender (Lavandula angustifolia)			X	X	X	X		X	X	X			X	X		X	X			X	X
Lemon (Citrus limon)					X				X				X	X						X	X
Lemongrass* (Cymbopogon citratus)			X		X													X			
Mandarin (Citrus reticulata)					X								X				X	X			
Marjoram, Spanish (Thymus mastichina)		X																			
Marjoram, sweet (Origanum majorana)		X	X		X	X		X	X	X		X	X	X		X	X	X	X	X	X
Melissa, True (Melissa officinalis)		X	X		X	X			X				X	X					X	X	X
Myrrh (Commiphora myrrha)				X	X	X															
Neroli (Citrus aurantium v. amara flos)			X		X			X			X	X				X	X	X		X	
Niaouli (Melaleuca viridiflora)				X			X		X												
Nutmeg* (Myristica fragrans)	X				X																
Orange, bitter (Citrus aurantium v. amara per)			X					X			X									X	
Orange, sweet (Citrus aurantium v. sinensis)			X					X			X										
Patchouli (Pogostemon patchouli)																					
Peppermint (Mentha x piperita)	X		X		X			X		X	X	X	X	X		X	X	X		X	X
Petitgrain (Citrus aurantium v. amara fol)					X			X		X									X		
Pine (Pinus sylvestris)	X		X		X		X	X		X									X	X	
Rose Otto (Rosa centifolia)	X		X		X			X		X	X								X	X	
Rosemary (Rosmarinus officinalis)	X	X	X				X	X			X	X	X	X		X	X		X	X	
Rosewood (Aniba rosaeodora)	X				X	X		X	X		X		X	X							
Sage (Salvia officinalis)	X	X			X	X		X	X												
Sandalwood (Santalum album)					X			X		X		X	X			X	X		X	X	
Savory* (Satureia montana)	X	X						X		X						X					
Tagetes (Tagetes glandulifera)	X		X																		
Tea Tree (Melaleuca alternifolia)	X			X			X	X		X		X			X		X	X		X	
Thyme* (Thymus vulgaris – phenols)					X			X		X		X									
Thyme, sweet (Thymus vulgaris – alcohols)	X	X	X	X	X			X	X	X		X	X			X		X		X	
Valerian (Valeriana officinalis)					X	X		X				X									
Vetiver (Vetiveria zizanioides)			X		X																
Ylang Ylang (Cananga odorata)					X			X		X	X	X									

* = should not be available to the general public

SKIN

Condition	Aniseed* (Pimpinella anisum)	Basil (sweet) (Ocimum basilicum)	Benzoin (Styrax benzoin)	Bergamot (Citrus bergamia)	Black Pepper (Piper nigrum)	Cajuput (Melaleuca leucadendron)	Camphor Wood (Cinnamomum camphora)	Caraway (Carum carvi)	Cedarwood (Cedrus atlantica)	Chamomile, German (Chamomilla recutita)	Chamomile, Moroccan (Ormenis mixta)	Chamomile, Roman (Chamaemelum nobile)	Cinnamon Bark* (Cinnamomum zerum)	Clary (Salvia sclarea)	Clove Bud* (Syzygium aromaticum)	Coriander (Coriandrum sativum)	Cypress (Cupressus sempervirens)	Dill (Anethum graveolens)	Eucalyptus (Eucalyptus globulus)	Fennel (Foeniculum vulgare)	Frankincense (Boswellia carteri)	Geranium (Pelargonium graveolens)	Ginger (Zingiber officinale)	Grapefruit (Citrus paradisi)	Hyssop* (Hyssopus officinalis)	Juniper (Juniperus communis)	Juniperberry (Juniperus communis)
Wrinkles (mature skin)														X								X		X			
Verrucae																											
Ulcers			X											X												X	
Thread Veins														X			X					X					
Sunburn																						X		X			
Stretch Marks																						X		X			
Sensitive														X													
Scars													X									X				X	
Psoriasis			X	X		X																					
Irritation													X	X													
Insect Bites	X					X																					
Inflammation														X					X			X	X				
Herpes				X	X													X				X					
Greasy (open pores)				X			X		X								X					X					
Eczema						X				X	X			X								X			X	X	X
Dry										X		X										X			X	X	X
Dermatitis			X	X		X				X	X								X			X			X	X	X
Cuts/Wounds			X	X		X				X			X						X			X			X		X
Cracked/Chapped			X			X																					
Burns			X			X				X												X					
Bruises							X			X									X						X		
Athlete's Foot																											
Acne			X			X			X	X				X								X					X
Abscesses/Boils						X				X				X													X

Lavandin (Lavandula x intermedia)

Lavender (Lavandula angustifolia)

Lemon (Citrus limon)

Lemongrass* (Cymbopogon citratus)

Mandarin (Citrus reticulata)

Marjoram, Spanish (Thymus mastichina)

Marjoram, sweet (Origanum majorana)

Melissa, True (Melissa officinalis)

Myrrh (Commiphora myrrha)

Neroli (Citrus aurantium v. amara flos)

Niaouli (Melaleuca viridiflora)

Nutmeg* (Myristica fragrans)

Orange, bitter (Citrus aurantium v. amara per)

Orange, sweet (Citrus aurantium v. sinensis)

Patchouli (Pogostemon patchouli)

Peppermint (Mentha x piperita)

Petitgrain (Citrus aurantium v. amara fol)

Pine (Pinus sylvestris)

Rose Otto (Rosa centifolia)

Rosemary (Rosmarinus officinalis)

Rosewood (Aniba rosaeodora)

Sage (Salvia officinalis)

Sandalwood (Santalum album)

Savory* (Satureia montana)

Tagetes (Tagetes glandulifera)

Tea Tree (Melaleuca alternifolia)

Thyme* (Thymus vulgaris – phenols)

Thyme, sweet (Thymus vulgaris – alcohols)

Valerian (Valeriana officinalis)

Vetiver (Vetiveria zizanioides)

Ylang ylang (Cananga odorata)

* = should not be available to the general public

	Insect Repellent	Air Disinfectant	Toothache	Sinusitis	Laryngitis	Infections	Gum Infections	Flu	Earache	Coughs/Colds	Catarrh	Bronchitis	Asthma
Aniseed* (*Pimpinella anisum*)												X	X
Basil (sweet) (*Ocimum basilicum*)	X			X					X				
Benzoin (*Styrax benzoin*)											X		
Bergamot (*Citrus bergamia*)													
Black Pepper (*Piper nigrum*)			X		X			X		X	X	X	X
Cajuput (*Melaleuca leucadendron*)			X	X	X			X	X		X	X	X
Camphor Wood (*Cinnamomum camphora*)													
Caraway (*Carum carvi*)												X	
Cedarwood (*Cedrus atlantica*)	X									X	X		
Chamomile, German (*Chamomilla recutita*)													X
Chamomile, Moroccan (*Ormenis mixta*)													
Chamomile, Roman (*Chamaemelum nobile*)			X						X				X
Cinnamon Bark* (*Cinnamomum verum*)							X						
Clary (*Salvia sclarea*)													
Clove Bud* (*Syzygium aromaticum*)	X		X	X			X					X	
Coriander (*Coriandrum sativum*)								X					
Cypress (*Cupressus sempervirens*)					X		X			X		X	
Dill (*Anethum graveolens*)													X
Eucalyptus (*Eucalyptus globulus*)	X	X		X	X			X		X		X	X
Fennel (*Foeniculum vulgare*)						X						X	
Frankincense (*Boswellia carteri*)						X						X	X
Geranium (*Pelargonium graveolens*)	X						X			X		X	
Ginger (*Zingiber officinale*)			X	X								X	
Grapefruit (*Citrus paradisi*)													
Hyssop* (*Hyssopus officinalis*)	X											X	X
Juniper (*Juniperus communis*)		X		X									
Juniperberry (*Juniperus communis*)							X			X		X	X

Lavandin (*Lavandula x intermedia*)		X																
Lavender (*Lavandula angustifolia*)	X	X	X															
Lemon (*Citrus limon*)	X	X	X				X	X						X	X	
Lemongrass* (*Cymbopogon citratus*)																
Mandarin (*Citrus reticulata*)																
Marjoram, Spanish (*Thymus mastichina*)	X	X	X				X									
Marjoram, sweet (*Origanum majorana*)	X	X	X				X									
Melissa, True (*Melissa officinalis*)																
Myrrh (*Commiphora myrrha*)	X		X		X		X									
Neroli (*Citrus aurantium v. amara flos*)																
Niaouli (*Melaleuca viridiflora*)	X	X	X		X	X	X	X								
Nutmeg* (*Myristica fragrans*)									X							
Orange, bitter (*Citrus aurantium v. amara per*)																
Orange, sweet (*Citrus aurantium v. sinensis*)																
Patchouli (*Pogostemon patchouli*)																
Peppermint (*Mentha x piperita*)		X	X		X	X	X	X					X			
Petitgrain (*Citrus aurantium v. amara fol*)					X											
Pine (*Pinus sylvestris*)	X	X	X		X	X	X	X					X			
Rose Otto (*Rosa centifolia*)	X	X														
Rosemary (*Rosmarinus officinalis*)		X	X	X			X	X								
Rosewood (*Aniba rosaeodora*)				X	X											
Sage (*Salvia officinalis*)	X	X	X		X	X	X	X					X			
Sandalwood (*Santalum album*)	X				X	X										
Savory* (*Satureia montana*)	X															
Tagetes (*Tagetes glandulifera*)		X														
Tea Tree (*Melaleuca alternifolia*)	X	X	X	X	X	X	X									
Thyme* (*Thymus vulgaris – phenols*)	X			X												
Thyme, sweet (*Thymus vulgaris – alcohols*)	X	X	X	X	X	X	X									
Valerian (*Valeriana officinalis*)																
Vetiver (*Vetiveria zizanioides*)																
Ylang ylang (*Cananga odorata*)																

* = should not be available to the general public

Glossary

Abortifacient:	Agent which can cause a miscarriage.
Aromatology:	The study of essential oils for health.
Astringent:	Contracting bodily tissues.
Carminative:	Relieving flatulence (wind).
Chemotype:	Plant grown from cutting in order to propagate plant with known chemical constituent.
Chemovar:	Another name for chemotype (v. or var. = variety).
Cholagogue:	Stimulating flow of bile.
Cicatrisant:	Healing, promoting scar tissue formation.
Cohobation:	Water used for distillation re-directed into system, to be used repeatedly in a closed cycle.
Cytophylactic:	Encouraging cell regeneration.
Diuretic:	Stimulating the secretion of urine.
Emmenagogue:	Inducing menstruation.
Emulsion:	A fluid formed by the suspension of one liquid in another, e.g. oil and water.
Endothelium:	The tissues covering the inside surfaces of the body.
Epithelium:	The tissues covering the outside surfaces of the body.
Expectorant:	Aids removal of catarrh.
Fixed oil:	Non-volatile lubricating extract from seeds or nuts, e.g. sunflower oil or almond oil.

Galactogogue:	Bringing on the flow of milk.
Hepatic:	Tonic to the liver.
Hepatoxic:	Toxic to the liver.
Hypertension:	High blood pressure.
Hypertensive:	That which raises blood pressure.
Hypotension:	Low blood pressure.
Hypotensive:	Lowers blood pressure.
Hormonal:	Balances (or regulates) the body's hormone secretion.
Immunostimulant:	Stimulating the body's own natural defence system.
Lipolytic: ʼ	Breaks down fat.
Mucolytic:	Breaks down mucus.
Nervine:	Nerve tonic.
Neurotoxic:	Toxic to the nervous system.
Osmology:	The study of smell.
Phytotherapy:	Use of the whole plant, as well as the essential oil, to aid healing.
Probiotic:	That which favours the beneficial bacteria in the body, while inhibiting harmful microbes. Literally 'favouring life'; as opposed to anti-biotic, 'hostile to life'.
Psychoneuroimmunology:	The study of the inter-relationship and mental effects of the mind, nervous system and body's defence system.
Purgative:	Causes evacuation of the bowels.
Quencher:	Quenches; i.e. suppresses unwanted possible secondary effects.
Rubefacient:	Increases local circulation, making skin red.
Scarification:	Making a series of small cuts – a method of extracting essence from citrus fruit peel.
Sedative:	Producing a calming effect.
Spasmolytic:	Relieving muscle spasm or cramp.
Stimulant:	Having a rousing, uplifting effect on body and mind.

Sudorific: Inducing perspiration.

Synergy: Literally means 'working together'; the phenomenon that occurs when two or more substances used together give a more effective result than any one of the substances used alone.

Vasoconstrictive: Causes contraction of the blood vessels.

Vulnerary: Healing agent for cuts, wounds and sores.

References

Chapter 1

1. Guenther E 1948 *The essential oils* van Nostrand, New York Vol 5: p3
2. Price L 1996 'Hildegard of Bingen.' *The Aromatherapist* Vol 3(4): pp22–26
3. Schilcher H 1985 'Effects and side effects of essential oils.' In Baerheim Svendsen A, Scheffer J J C (eds) 1985 *Essential oils and aromatic plants* Martinus Nighoff/Dr W Junk Publishers, Dordrecht: p221

Chapter 2

4. Müller J, Bräuer H, Hersing J, Beck C 1984 *H & R Book of Perfume* Johnson, London: p73
5. Arctander S 1961 *Perfume and flavor materials of natural origin* Self published, Elizabeth, New Jersey: p34
6. Arctander S 1961 *Perfume and flavor materials of natural origin* Self published, Elizabeth, New Jersey: p311
7. Müller, J, Bräuer H, Hersing J, Beck C 1984 *H & R Book of Perfume* Johnson, London: p111
8a. Guenther E 1948 *The essential oils* van Nostrand, New York Vol 1: p219
8b. Guenther E 1948 *The essential oils* van Nostrand, New York Vol 1: p220
8c. Guenther E 1948 *The essential oils* van Nostrand, New York Vol 1: p178
9. Opdyke D L J 1976 'Inhibition of sensitization reactions induced by certain aldehydes,' *Food and Cosmetics Toxicology* 14(3): pp197–198

Chapter 3

10. Witty D 1993 (personal communication)
11. Price S, Price L 1999 *Aromatherapy for health professionals* (revised 2nd edition) Churchill Livingstone, Edinburgh: p27

12. Price L 1990 Aromatherapy course notes. Shirley Price International College of Aromatherapy, Hinckley

13. Buchbauer G 1993 'Biological effects of fragrances and essential oils'. *Perfumer & Flavorist* 18: p22

14. Price S, Price L 1999 *Aromatherapy for health professionals* (revised 2nd edition) Churchill Livingstone, Edinburgh: p52

15. Franchomme P, Pénoël D 1990 *L'aromathérapie exactement* Jollois, Limoges: pp93–100

Chapter 4

16. Durrafourd P 1982 *En forme tous les jours* La Vie Claire, Périgny: p102

17. Guenther E 1948 *The essential oils* van Nostrand, New York Vol 5: p278

18. Tisserand R, Balacs T 1995 *Essential oil safety* Churchill Livingstone, Edinburgh: p186

19. Arctander S 1961 *Perfume and flavor materials of natural origin* Self published, Elizabeth, New Jersey: p241

20. Schnaubelt K 1992 Aromatherapy correspondence course notes

21. Arctander S 1961 *Perfume and flavor materials of natural origin* Self published, Elizabeth, New Jersey: p387

22. Grieve M 1998 *A modern herbal* Tiger Books International, Twickenham

23. Mabey R (ed.) 1988 *The complete new herbal* Elm Tree Books, London: p122

24. Lawrence B M 1980 'Progress in essential oils' *Perfumer & Flavorist* 5(4): p33

25. Tisserand R, Balacs T 1995 *Essential oil safety* Churchill Livingstone, Edinburgh: pp157–158

26. Mabey R (ed.) 1988 *The complete new herbal* Elm Tree Books, London: p121

27. Franchomme P, Pénoël D 1990 *L'aromathérapie exactement* Jollois, Limoges: p384

28. Lawless J 1992 *The encyclopaedia of essential oils* Element, Shaftesbury: p175

29. Price S, Price L 1999 *Aromatherapy for health professionals* (revised 2nd edition) Churchill Livingstone, Edinburgh: p315

30. Franchomme P, Pénoël D 1990 *L'aromathérapie exactement* Jollois, Limoges: p342

31. Arctander S 1961 *Perfume and flavor materials of natural origin* Self published, Elizabeth, New Jersey: p210

32. Mabey R (ed.) 1988 *The complete new herbal* Elm Tree Books, London

33. Lautié R and Passebecq A 1979 *Aromatherapy* Thorsons, Wellingborough: p37

34. Franchomme P, Pénoël D 1990 *L'aromathérapie exactement* Jollois, Limoges: p359

35. Tisserand R, Balacs T 1995 *Essential oil safety* Churchill Livingstone, Edinburgh: p140

36. Lamy M 1990 Lecture notes. Chambre d'Agriculture, Nyons

37. Leicester R J, Hunt R H 1982 'Peppermint oil to reduce colonic spasm during endoscopy' *The Lancet*, 30 October: p989

38. Price S, Price L 1999 *Aromatherapy for health professionals* (revised 2nd edition) Churchill Livingstone, Edinburgh: p333

39. Franchomme P, Pénoël D 1990 *L'aromathérapie exactement* Jollois, Limoges: p375

40. Opdyke D L J 1978 'Spearmint oil' *Food and Cosmetics Toxicology* Vol 16 Special Issue 4: p871

41. Battaglia S 1995 *The complete guide to aromatherapy* The Perfect Potion, Virginia: p179

42. Price S 1999 *Practical Aromatherapy* (revised 4th edition) Thorsons, London: p177

43. Tisserand R, Balacs T 1995 *Essential oil safety* Churchill Livingstone, Edinburgh: p209

44. Durrafourd P 1982 *En forme tous les jours* La Vie Claire, Périgny: p107

45. Franchomme P, Pénoël D 1990 *L'aromathérapie exactement* Jollois, Limoges: p394

46. Price S, Price L 1999 *Aromatherapy for health professionals* (revised 2nd edition) Churchill Livingstone, Edinburgh: p342

47. Roulière G 1990 *Les huiles essentielles pour votre santé* Dangles, St-Jean-de-Braye: p302

48. Battaglia S 1995 *The complete guide to aromatherapy* The Perfect Potion, Virginia: p156

49. Deans S G, Svoboda K P 1989 'Antibacterial activity of summer savory (*Satureia hortensis*) essential oil and its constituents' *Journal of Horticultural Science* 64: pp205–211

50. Franchomme P, Pénoël D 1990 *L'aromathérapie exactement* Jollois, Limoges: p401

51. Price S 1999 *Practical Aromatherapy* (revised 4th edition) Thorsons, London: p152

52. Henglein M 1991 Lecture notes. Shirley Price International College of Aromatherapy, Hinckley

53. Roulière G 1990 *Les huiles essentielles pour votre santé* Dangles, St-Jean-de-Braye: p243

54. Franchomme P, Pénoël D 1990 *L'aromathérapie exactement* Jollois, Limoges: p335

55. Pénoël D 1992 (personal communication)

56. Franchomme P, Pénoël D 1990 *L'aromathérapie exactement* Jollois, Limoges: p369

57. Arctander S 1961 *Perfume and flavor materials of natural origin* Self published, Elizabeth, New Jersey: p110

58. Franchomme P, Pénoël D 1990 *L'aromathérapie exactement* Jollois, Limoges: p370

59. Mailhebiau P 1994 *La Nouvelle Aromathérapie* Jakin, Lausanne: p427

60. Arctander S 1961 *Perfume and flavor materials of natural origin* Self published, Elizabeth, New Jersey: p311

61. Durrafourd P 1982 *En forme tous les jours* La Vie Claire, Périgny: p78

62. Guenther E 1948 *The essential oils* van Nostrand, New York Vol 5: p5

63. Secondini O 1990 *Handbook of perfume and flavors* Chemical Publishing, New York: p408

64. Wabner D 1992 (personal communication)

65. Price S, Price L 1999 *Aromatherapy for health professionals* (revised 2nd edition) Churchill Livingstone, Edinburgh: p341

66. Mailhebiau P 1994 *La Nouvelle Aromathérapie* Jakin, Lausanne: p283

67. Guenther E 1948 *The essential oils* van Nostrand, New York Vol 3: p264

68. Price S, Price L 1999 *Aromatherapy for health professionals* (revised 2nd edition) Churchill Livingstone, Edinburgh: p321

69. Roulière G 1990 *Les huiles essentielles pour votre santé* Dangles, St-Jean-de-Braye: p292

70. Franchomme P, Pénoël D 1990 *L'aromathérapie exactement* Jollois, Limoges: p324

71. Guenther E 1948 *The essential oils* van Nostrand, New York Vol 6: p264

Chapter 5

72. Opdyke D L J 1973 'Basil oil, sweet' *Food and Cosmetics Toxicology* Vol 11: p86

73. Franchomme P, Pénoël D 1990 *L'aromathérapie exactement* Jollois, Limoges: p380

74. Tisserand R, Balacs T 1991 Research reports. *International Journal of Aromatherapy* Vol 3(1): p6

75. Guenther E 1948 *The essential oils* van Nostrand, New York Vol 4: p260

76. Pénoël D 1993 (personal communication)

77. Tisserand R, Balacs T 1995 *Essential oil safety* Churchill Livingstone, Edinburgh: p204

78. Arctander S 1961 *Perfume and flavor materials of natural origin* Self published, Elizabeth, New Jersey: p140

79. Schilcher H 1984 Lecture notes. 15th symposium in essential oils

80. Arctander S 1961 *Perfume and flavor materials of natural origin* Self published, Elizabeth, New Jersey: p109

81. Guenther E 1948 *The essential oils* van Nostrand, New York Vol 6: p389

82. Wren R C 1975 *Potter's new cyclopaedia of botanical drugs and preparations* Health Science Press, Hengiscote

83. Arctander S 1961 *Perfume and flavor materials of natural origin* Self published, Elizabeth, New Jersey: p157

84. Price L 1998 'Moroccan wild chamomile' *Aromatherapy World* Summer: pp14–15

85. Opdyke D L J 1975 'Eucalyptus oil' *Food and Cosmetics Toxicology* Vol 13: p107

86. Guenther E 1948 *The essential oils* van Nostrand, New York Vol 4: p671

87. Guenther E 1948 *The essential oils* van Nostrand, New York Vol 6: pp374–5

88. Lamy M 1990 Lecture notes. Chambre d'Agriculture, Nyons

89. Price L 1994 Lavenders and lavandins. Lecture notes. Shirley Price International College of Aromatherapy, Hinckley

90. Arctander S 1961 *Perfume and flavor materials of natural origin* Self published, Elizabeth, New Jersey: p401

91. Franchomme P, Pénoël D 1990 *L'aromathérapie exactement* Jollois, Limoges: pp383–384

92. Mailhebiau P 1994 *La Nouvelle Aromathérapie* Jakin, Lausanne: p165

93. Arctander S 1961 *Perfume and flavor materials of natural origin* Self published, Elizabeth, New Jersey: p493

94. Arctander S 1961 *Perfume and flavor materials of natural origin* Self published, Elizabeth, New Jersey: p211

95. Arctander S 1961 *Perfume and flavor materials of natural origin* Self published, Elizabeth, New Jersey: p485

96. Guenther E 1948 *The essential oils* van Nostrand, New York Vol 3: p640

97. Arctander S 1961 *Perfume and flavor materials of natural origin* Self published, Elizabeth, New Jersey: pp412–415

98. Poucher W A 1979 *Perfumes, cosmetics & soaps* Chapman and Hall, London: p298

99. Franchomme P, Pénoël D 1990 *L'aromathérapie exactement* Jollois, Limoges: p388

100. Henglein M 1991 Lecture notes. Shirley Price International College of Aromatherapy, Hinckley

101. Poucher W A 1979 *Perfumes, cosmetics & soaps* Chapman and Hall, London: p328

102. Arctander S 1961 *Perfume and flavor materials of natural origin* Self published, Elizabeth, New Jersey: p102

103. Price S 1999 *Practical Aromatherapy* (revised 4th edition) Thorsons, London: p153

104. Battaglia S 1995 *The complete guide to aromatherapy* The Perfect Potion, Virginia: pp207–208

105. Arctander S 1961 *Perfume and flavor materials of natural origin* Self published, Elizabeth, New Jersey: pp669–671

106. Battaglia S 1995 *The complete guide to aromatherapy* The Perfect Potion, Virginia: p52

Chapter 6

107. Verdet D 1991 Lecture notes. Shirley Price International College of Aromatherapy French field study trip, Sainte Croix

108. Pénoël D 1992 (personal communication)

109. Witty D 1992 (personal communication)

110. Price S, Price L 1999 *Aromatherapy for health professionals* (revised 2nd edition) Churchill Livingstone, Edinburgh: p177

111. Wabner D 1993 (personal communication)

112. Valette C 1945 Comptes rendus 13 Oct cited in: Anon. 1947 'Pénétration transcutanée des essences' *Parfümerie Modern* 39: pp64–66

113. Bennett G 1992 The reticuloendothelial system. Lecture notes. Shirley Price International College of Aromatherapy, Hinckley

Chapter 7

114. Günther Ohloff 1990 *Reichstoffe und Geruchsinn* Springer-Verlag, Berlin
115. Brun K 1952 *Les essences végétales en tant qu'agent de pénétration tissulaire* Thèse Pharmacie, Strasbourg
116. Valnet J 1980 *The practice of aromatherapy* Daniel, Saffron Walden: p26
117. Low D, Rawal B D, Griffin W J 1974 Antibacterial action of the essential oils of some Australian Myrtaceae with special references to the activity of chromatographic fractions of oil of *Eucalyptus citriodora. Planta Medica* 26: pp184–189

Chapter 8

118. Valette G, Sobrin E 1963 'Percutaneous absorption of various animal and vegetable oils' *Pharmaceutica Acta Helvetica* 39 (1–6): p64
119. Leung A Y, Foster S 1996 *Encyclopaedia of common natural ingredients used in food, drugs and cosmetics* Wiley, New York: pp22–23
120. Monograph 1986 'Calendula flos' *Bundesanzeiger*, 13 March no. 50
121. Bruneton J 1995 *Pharmacognancy, phytomedicine, medicinal plants* Intercept, Andover: pp562–563
122. Price L 1999 *Carrier oils for aromatherapy and massage* (revised 3rd edition) Riverhead, Stratford upon Avon: p53
123. Winter R 1984 *A consumer's dictionary of cosmetic ingredients* Crown, New York: p73
124. Bartram T 1996 *Encyclopaedia of herbal medicine* Grace, Christchurch: p175
125. Graham J 1984 *Evening primrose oil* Thorsons, Wellingborough: pp45–85
126. Ferrando J 1986 'Clinical trial of topical application containing urea, sunflower oil, evening primrose oil, wheatgerm oil and sodium pyruvate, in several hyperkeratotic skin conditions' *Med Cutan Lat Am* 14(2): pp132–137
127. Winter R 1984 *A consumer's dictionary of cosmetic ingredients* Crown, New York: p127
128. Earle L *Vital oils* Ebury Press, London: p116
129. INTEC 1992 'Gathering and industrialisation of Chilean hazelnut oil' Report sponsored by the Agricultural Planning Office (ODEPA): p13
130. Price L 1999 *Carrier oils for aromatherapy and massage* (revised 3rd edition) Riverhead, Stratford upon Avon: p133
131. Bruneton J 1995 *Pharmacognancy, phytomedicine, medicinal plants* Intercept, Andover: pp367–368
132. Bartram T 1996 *Encyclopaedia of herbal medicine* Grace, Christchurch: p258
133. de Boeck W 1992 (personal communication)
134. Earle L 1995 *Quick guides: food allergies* Boxtree, London: p28
135. Price L 1999 *Carrier oils for aromatherapy and massage* (revised 3rd edition) Riverhead, Stratford upon Avon

136. Mabey R (ed.) 1988 *The complete new herbal* Elm Tree Books, London: p14
137. Sanecki K 1987 'The domestic and cosmetic use of herbs' In: Stuart M (ed.) 1987 *The encyclopedia of herbs and herbalism* Black Cat, London: pp108–109

Chapter 9

138. Bennett G 1992 *Handbook of clinical dietetics* Price Publishing, Stratford upon Avon: p20
139. Price S, Price L 1999 *Aromatherapy for health professionals* (revised 2nd edition) Churchill Livingstone, Edinburgh: p3
140. Franchomme P, Pénoël D 1990 *L'aromathérapie exactement* Jollois, Limoges: p402
141. Valnet J 1980 *The practice of aromatherapy* Daniel, Saffron Walden: pp87 & 92
142. Lawless J 1992 *The encyclopaedia of essential oils* Element, Shaftesbury: p54
143. Anon. 1991 'Placebo power: your mind and how it heals you' *Here's Health* October: p20
144. *British Medical Journal* 1884: 1: p1163
145. Bennett G 1990 Teacher training lecture notes. Shirley Price International College of Aromatherapy, Hinckley
146. Bennett G 1992 *Handbook of clinical dietetics* Price Publishing, Stratford upon Avon: p66

Chapter 10

147. Anckett A 1979 'Baby massage alternative to drugs' *Australian Nursing Journal* 9(5): pp24–27
148. Beard G, Wood E C 1964 *Massage principles and techniques* Saunders, Philadelphia: p56
149. Chaitow L 1987 *Soft tissue manipulation* Thorsons, Wellingborough: p22
150. Beard G, Wood E C 1964 *Massage principles and techniques*, Saunders, Philadelphia: p38
151. Cawthorne A 1991 'Aromatherapy on trial' *Aromanews* 30: pp7–8

Chapter 11

152. Price S, Price L 1999 *Aromatherapy for health professionals* (revised 2nd edition) Churchill Livingstone, Edinburgh: p80
153. Battaglia S 1995 *The complete guide to aromatherapy* The Perfect Potion, Virginia: p195
154. Grant E *The bitter pill* Corgi Books, Reading: p34
155. Grant E *The bitter pill* Corgi Books, Reading: p101
156. Price S, Price L 1999 *Aromatherapy for health professionals* (revised 2nd edition) Churchill Livingstone, Edinburgh: p177
157. Price S 1991 *Aromatherapy for common ailments* Gaia Books, London: p5
158. Price P 1996 *Pregnancy monograph* Shirley Price International College of Aromatherapy, Hinckley
159. Price S, Price-Parr P 1996 *Aromatherapy for babies and children* Thorsons, London: p63
160. Price S, Price-Parr P 1996 *Aromatherapy for babies and children* Thorsons, London: p106

Chapter 12

161. Deans S G, Svoboda K P 1989 'Antibacterial activity of summer savory (*Satureia hortensis*) essential oil and its constituents' *Journal of Horticultural Science* 64: pp205–211

162. Valnet J 1980 *The practice of aromatherapy* Daniel, Saffron Walden: pp34–35

163. Schilcher H 1985 'Effects and side effects of essential oils' In: Baerheim Svendsen A, Scheffer J J C (eds) 1985 *Essential oils and aromatic plants* Martinus Nijihoff/Dr W Junk Publishers, Dordrecht: p221

164. Durrafourd P 1982 *En forme tous les jours* La Vie Claire, Périgny: p87

165. Price L 1990 Aromatherapy course notes. Shirley Price International College of Aromatherapy, Hinckley

Further Reading

Davis P 1988 *Aromatherapy – An A–Z*, Daniel, Saffron Walden
Earle L 1991 *Vital Oils*, Ebury Press, London
Hay L L 1987 *You Can Heal Your Life*, Eden Grove, London
Lawless J 1992 *Encyclopaedia of Essential Oils*, Element Books, Shaftesbury
Price S 1991 *Aromatherapy for Common Ailments*, Gaia Books, London
Price S 1999 *Practical Aromatherapy* (4th edition), Thorsons, London
Price S 2000 *Aromatherapy for Your Emotions*, Thorsons, London
Price S, Price L 1999 *Aromatherapy for Health Professionals* (2nd edition), Churchill Livingstone, Edinburgh
Price S, Price-Parr P 1996 *Aromatherapy for Babies and Children*, Thorsons, London
Sanderson H, Harrison J, Price S 1993 *Aromatherapy for People With Learning Difficulties*, Hands on Publishing, Birmingham
Stanway P 1989 *Diets for Common Ailments*, Gaia Books, London
Thomas S 1989 *Massage for Common Ailments*, Gaia Books, London
Tisserand M 1990 *Aromatherapy for Women*, Thorsons, London
Tisserand R 1988 *Aromatherapy for Everyone*, Penguin Books, Middlesex
Valnet J 1980 *Practice of Aromatherapy*, Daniel, Saffron Walden
Wood C 1990 *Say Yes to Life*, Dent, London
Worwood V 1990 *The Fragrant Pharmacy*, Macmillan, London

Useful Addresses

Aromatherapy products

Great Britain
Shirley Price Aromatherapy Ltd
Essentia House
Upper Bond Street
Hinckley
Leics LE10 1RS
Tel: 01455 615466
Fax: 01455 615054

Herbal Garden
20 Eldon Gardens
Percy Street
Newcastle
Tyne & Wear

Herbal Garden
93 Rose Street
Edinburgh
Lothian EH2 3DT

Training
Aromatherapy

Shirley Price International College
  of Aromatherapy Ltd
Address as above
Tel: 01455 633231

The S.E.E.D. Institute
Therapeutic Division
10 Magnolia Way
Fleet
Hants GU13 9JZ

Aromatherapy and specialized short courses
Penny Price
Sketchley Manor
Burbage
Leics LE10 2LQ
Fax: 01455 617972

Aromatic medicine and aromatology
Robert Stephen (consultant)
4 Woodland Road
Hinckley
Leics LE10 1JG
Tel/Fax: 01455 611829

Aromatic medicine association
The Institute of Aromatic Medicine (IAM)
Aromed House
41 Leicester Road
Hinckley
Leics LE10 1LW

Aromatherapy Associations

Aromatherapy Organisations Council
  (AOC)
PO Box 19834
London SE25 6WF
Tel: 020 8251 7912
Fax: 010 8251 7942

International Society of Professional
  Aromatherapists (ISPA)
ISPA House
82 Ashby Road
Hinckley
Leics LE10 1SN
Tel: 01455 647987
Fax: 01455 890956

International Federation of
  Aromatherapists (IFA)
Stamford House
2/4 Chiswick High Street
London W4 1TH
Tel: 020 8742 2605
Fax: 020 8742 2606

Aromatherapy training and products

Australia
Australian School of Awareness
PO Box 187
Montrose
Victoria 3765
Australia
Tel: (03) 9723 2509
Fax: (03) 9761 8895

Israel
Fern Allen
PO Box 4363
Jerusalem
Israel
Tel: 00 972 267 9908

Italy
Jenny Bird
Via Vigevano 43
Milan 20144
Italy
Tel: 00 39 258 113261

Northern Ireland
European College of Natural Therapies
16 North Parade
Belfast BT7 2GG
Northern Ireland
Tel: 01232 641454

Republic of Ireland
Mary Cavanagh
Chamomile
Three Mile Water
Wicklow
Eire
Tel: 00 353 404 47219
Fax: 00 353 404 47319

Christine Courtney
Oban Aromatherapy
53 Beech Grove
Lucan
Co. Dublin
Eire
Tel: 00 353 1628 2121

Norway
Margareth Thomte
Nedreslottsgate 25
0157 Oslo
Norway
Tel: 00 47 22 170017
Fax: 00 47 22 425777

Switzerland
Sara Gelzer
Eigentalstr 552 No 14
8425 Oberembrach
Switzerland
Tel: 00 41 1 865 4996

USA

Training and products

Nordblom Swedish Healthcare Centre
178 Mill Creek Road
Livingstone
Montana 59047
USA
Tel: 001 406 333 4216
Fax: 001 406 333 4415

Training

The Australasian College of Herbal Studies
PO Box 57
Lake Oswego
Oregon 97034
USA
Tel: 001 503 635 6652
Fax: 001 503 697 0615

R J Buckle Associates
PO Box 868
Hunter
NY 12442
USA
Tel: 001 518 263 4405
Fax: 001 518 263 4031

Aromatherapy Association

National Association for Holistic
   Aromatherapy
PO Box 17622
Boulder
Colorado 80308 – 7622
USA
Tel: 001 888–ASK–NAHA
Tel: 001 314 963 2071
Fax: 001 314 963 4454

Stockists only

Northern Ireland
Angela Hillis
32 Russell Park
Belfast
Co. Antrim BT5 7QW
Northern Ireland

Iceland
Bergfell ehf
Skipholt 50c
105 Reykjavik
Iceland
Tel: 00 354 551 5060
Fax: 00 354 551 5065

Japan
Oz International Ltd
K5 Building
6F 4–5 Kojimachi
Chiyodaku
Tokyo 102–0083
Japan
Tel: 00 81 3 5213 3060
Fax: 00 81 3 3262 1970

Korea
Jung Dong Cosmetics Co Ltd
501 Shinham Officetel
49-5 Chungdam-Dong
Kangnam-Ku
Seoul
Korea

Malta
Professional Health & Beauty Services
Comflor APT
1B Marfa Road
Mellieha Bay
SPB10 Malta

Singapore
Eden Marketing Pte
63 Hillview Avenue
09-21 Lam Soon Industrial Building
Singapore 2366
Tel: 00 65 7696168
Fax: 00 65 7693937

Taiwan
Chun Hun
8F, No 205, Sec. 1
Fu-Shin S. Road
Taipei
Taiwan
Tel: 00 886 2751 3590
Fax: 00 886 2776 3547/1599

Jong Yeong Cosmetics Co Ltd
16 Tze Chyang 3rd Road
Nan Kang Industry Park
Nan Tou
Taiwan
Tel: 00 886 49 251065
Fax: 00 886 49 251071

Index

Guildford College
Learning Resource Centre

Please return on or before the last date shown
This item may be renewed by telephone unless overdue

Class: _615. 32 PRI_

Title: _Aromatherapy Workbook_

Author: _PRICE, Shirley_